Herbal Immunity Boosters Against COVID-19

Edited By

Sachin Kumar Jain
Oriental College of Pharmacy & Research
Oriental University
MP-452010
India

Ram Kumar Sahu
Department of Pharmaceutical Science
Sushruta School of Medical and Paramedical Sciences
Assam University (A Central University)
Silchar-788011, Assam
India

Priyanka Soni
B R Nahata College of Pharmacy
Mandsaur University,
Mandsaur Assam
India

&

Vishal Soni
B R Nahata College of Pharmacy
Mandsaur University,
Mandsaur Assam
India

Herbal Immunity Boosters Against COVID-19

Editors: Sachin Kumar Jain, Ram Kumar Sahu, Priyanka Soni & Vishal Soni

ISBN (Online): 978-981-5079-45-6

ISBN (Print): 978-981-5079-46-3

ISBN (Paperback): 978-981-5079-47-0

First published in 2022.

Bentham Science Publishers Pte. Ltd.
80 Robinson Road #02-00
Singapore 068898
Singapore
Email: subscriptions@benthamscience.net

BENTHAM SCIENCE

CONTENTS

PREFACE

The book is an exclusive version of the instructive matter on Herbal Immunity Boosters for Covid-19. The herbal immunity booster is basically an emerging field that discusses potential preparations to diminish the severity of the infection caused by Covid-19. Currently, the effective treatment of COVID-19 is lacking. Hence it is imperative for individuals to use such type of food supplements which boost their immune systems. In this concern, the ideal technique is to fortify immunity naturally by using medicinal plants. Whereas, immunity booster deals with the remarkable protection mechanism against loads of bacteria, viruses, fungi, toxins and parasites when entering the body. Additionally, other signaling pathways are recognized that are responsible for the regulation of the pathogenesis of infections and non-infectious diseases due to lower immunity. It also deals with the exploration of functional and nutraceutical foods for preserving body homeostasis which is essential to maintain immunity. Therefore, plants or herbs having immunomodulating properties should be included in the diet, and we should explore novel therapeutic opportunities to improve immunity against diseases. This book contains immense knowledge about Herbal Immunity Boosters for Covid-19 with respect to the mode of action, modulation of signaling pathways, regulatory aspects, safety, food supplements and drug delivery for better function of the immune system. In addition, drug development issues, adaptation to clinical use, market prospects and industrial commercialization too come under the concept of Herbal Immunity Boosters for Covid-19. The book not only focuses on theoretical knowledge but also considers practical aspects. The book is very beneficial for students and researchers across the globe that are indulged in the reading and investigation of Herbal Immunity Boosters for Covid-19, thereby, spreading awareness all over the globe and promoting anticipated trends in the field of Herbal Immunity Boosters. The major objective of this initiative is to bring into light the entire fundamental concept. This book also includes different types of procedures and herbal medicines to increase and treatment and immunity of Covid-19.

Sachin Kumar Jain
Oriental College of Pharmacy & Research Oriental University
Ujjain Road Indore MP-452010
India

Ram Kumar Sahu
Department of Pharmaceutical Science
Sushruta School of Medical and Paramedical Sciences
Assam University (A Central University)
Silchar-788011
Assam, India

Priyanka Soni
B R Nahata College of Pharmacy
Mandsaur University,
Mandsaur Assam
India

&

Vishal Soni
B R Nahata College of Pharmacy
Mandsaur University,
Mandsaur Assam
India

List of Contributors

Ankit Jain	IPS Academy College of Pharmacy, Rajendra Nagar AB Road, Indore MP, India
Aseem Setia	Department of Pharmaceutics, ISF College of Pharmacy, Moga, Punjab-142001, India
Chayanika Bordoloi	NEF College of Pharmacy, Guwahati, Assam, India
Deepshikha Verma	Institute of Pharmaceutical Sciences, Guru Ghasidas Vishwavidyalaya, Koni, Bilaspur-495009, Chhattisgarh, India
Km. Nandani Jayaswal	Department of Pharmaceutics, ISF College of Pharmacy, Moga, Punjab-142001, India
Lubhan Singh	KSCP, Swami Vivekanand Subharti University, Meerut, Uttar Pradesh, India
Neetesh Kumar Jain	Faculty of Pharmacy, Oriental University Indore, MP, India
Nitu Singh	Faculty of Pharmacy, Oriental University Indore, MP, India
Priyanka Pandey	Swami Vivekanand College of Pharmacy, Indore, Madhya Pradesh, India
Ram Kumar Sahu	Department of Pharmaceutical Science, Assam University (A Central University), Silchar, Assam – 788011, India
Raja Chakraborty	Institute of Pharmacy, Assam Don Bosco University, Tepesia Garden, Sonapur, India
Rakesh Sagar	Department of Pharmacy SGSITS, Indore MP, India
Ravindra Kumar Pandey	Columbia Institute of Pharmacy, Tekari, Raipur, Chhattisgarh, India
Retno Widyowati	Department of Pharmaceutical Science, Faculty of Pharmacy, Universitas Airlangga, Surabaya, 60115, Indonesia
Rupesh Kumar Pandey	KSCP, Swami Vivekanand Subharti University, Meerut, Uttar Pradesh, India
Saikat Sen	Faculty of Pharmaceutical Science, Assam Down Town University, Guwahati, Assam, India
Sachin Kumar Jain	Oriental College of Pharmacy & Research, Oriental University, Ujjain Road Indore MP-452010, India
Saket Singh Chandel	Department of Pharmacology, Dr. C. V. Raman Institute of Pharmacy, Dr. C. V. Raman University, Bilaspur-495113, Chhattisgarh, India
Shiv Shankar Shukla	Columbia Institute of Pharmacy, Tekari, Raipur, Chhattisgarh, India
Sokindra Kumar	KSCP, Swami Vivekanand Subharti University, Meerut, Uttar Pradesh, India
Sunil Mistry	Apex Institute of Pharmacy, Samaspur, Chunar, Mirzapur UP, India 231304
Upendra S. Bhadoriya	IPS Academy College of Pharmacy, Rajendra Nagar AB Road, Indore MP, India
Vinod Nautiyal	Department of Pharmaceutical Sciences, Gurukul Kangri University Haridwar, Uttarakhand, India

Vipinchandra Bhaskarrao Pande Department of Pharmacy, Mandsaur University, Mandsaur-458001, Madhya Pradesh, India

Vishal Trivedi Department of Pharmacy, Madhav University, Abu Road, Pindwara, Rajasthan, India

CHAPTER 1

Origin of COVID-19

Aseem Setia[1], **Km. Nandani Jayaswal**[1] and **Ram Kumar Sahu**[2,*]

[1] *Department of Pharmaceutics, ISF College of Pharmacy, Moga, Punjab-142001, India*

[2] *Department of Pharmaceutical Sciences, Assam University (A Central University), Silchar, Assam – 788011, India*

Abstract: Coronavirus is a type of virus that is surrounded by non-segmented, single-stranded, positive-sense RNA genomes that reproduce in the cytoplasm. The size of the coronavirus is usually 80-120 nm. It was discovered in Wuhan, China in December 2019, and it was termed 2019 nCoV or COVID-19. The coronavirus is encased in a lipid bilayer and it possesses several proteins. These proteins are surrounded in the envelope of a virus; whereas, in the viral RNA, N-protein shows interactions and it can be found on the outer surface of the viral particle, forming the nucleocapsid. The spike protein is identified as the leading protein and mediates the entrance inside the host body that would cause SARS-CoV-2syndrome. The spike protein has two spheres namely S1 and S2. The receptor that is attached to the S1 and further S2 is responsible for fusion. In the past, the most severe types of virus which had resulted in large-scale pandemics were SARS (in 2002–2003) which occurred in Guandong Province, China. Meanwhile, Saudi Arabia had experienced the Middle East respiratory syndrome (MERS) in 2012. The virus in the 1960s was commonly identified in birds and mammals; mostly in rats, camels, cats and bats. SARS-CoV-2 causative agents belong to the genus β-Coronavirus. Coronavirus can be classified into four genera such as α, β, γ, and δ coronavirus. Alpha and beta coronaviruses are found in mammals such as bats. Gamma coronaviruses would primarily infect birds and affect mammalians, whereas delta coronaviruses would infect both birds and mammals. This chapter highlights the origin, historical background, the classification of the coronavirus as well as providing the conceptual information on various treatment approaches for COVID-19.

Keywords: β-Coronavirus, Coronavirus, MERS-CoV, SARS-CoV, SARS-Co--2, Spike Protein.

1. INTRODUCTION

Coronavirus is a chief pathogen that principally infects the respiratory tract of humans. Previous coronavirus outbreaks (CoVs) have shown syndromes of the

* **Corresponding author Ram Kumar Sahu:** Department of Pharmaceutical Science, Assam University (A Central University), Silchar, Assam – 788011, India; E-mail: ramsahu79@gmail.com

Middle East respiratory syndrome (MERS)-CoV as well as a severe acute respiratory syndrome (SARS)-CoV. These syndromes were alarming to the world's population due to the infections they had caused [1]. SARS-CoV first appeared in 2002, followed by (MERS-CoV) and the novel coronavirus in 2012 and 2019, respectively. COVID-19, which was recently discovered, is the fifth known pandemic since the 1918 flu pandemic [2]. Coronaviruses are viruses enclosed with non-segmented, single-stranded, positive-sense RNA genomes that reproduce in the cytoplasm and they are typically 80-120 nm in size. COVID-19 was first identified in December 2019 in Wuhan, China, and was later referred to as 2019 nCoV or COVID-19 [3]. The SARS-CoV virus is a member of the Coronaviridae family, specifically the orthocoronaviridae subfamily and the order Nidovirales. The size range of the RNA genome lies between 26 to 32 kb. A helical nucleocapsid encompasses the DNA, which is surrounded by a lipid bilayer that is derived from the host [4]. Membrane (M), Spike (S), envelope (E) and nucleocapsid (N) are proteins found on the surface of the coronavirus (N). The S protein is the primary viral entry point [5]. The S protein is a large, Type-I transmembrane protein with 1160 amino acids for avian infectious bronchitis virus (IBV) and 1400 amino acids for feline coronavirus (FCoV). In the S protein, two domains namely S1 and S2 were discovered. The two domains S1 and S2 would recognize the host receptor and act for further fusion, respectively [6]. Once it is attached to the receptor, the envelop spike proteins would enter the host body directly through the cell surface and *via* the endocytosis fusion process. The massive conformational changes in the spike protein would determine the virus-host membrane fusion. Coronavirus has the appearance of a crown in an electron microscope and it is due to the presence of the glycoprotein spikes on its cover [7]. The MHV receptor was first discovered in 1991 and it was identified as the leading coronavirus binding receptor as it would allow the MHV to infect cells by binding them to the CEACAM1 molecule [8]. CEACAM1 is a part of the immunoglobulin superfamily and it is classified as a Type-I transmembrane protein. The multifunctional protein CEACAM1 plays a major role in the adhesion and cell signalling. Human coronaviruses consist of seven strains namely Human Coronavirus OC43 (HCoV-OC43), MERS-CoV, SARS-CoV (HCoV-NL63, New Heaven Coronavirus), Human Coronavirus HKU1, Human Coronavirus 229E (HCoV-229E), HCoV-EMC as well as the new strain that is identified as the Wuhan coronavirus which is known to be extremely dangerous and currently spreading widely worldwide (known as SARS-CoV-2 or COVID-19). Coronavirus Humanoid viruses, such as HCoV-229E, -NL63, -OC43 and –HKU1 are common in the humanoid population and they would display severe infection in the human respiratory tract at every age group. Alpha coronaviruses consist of HCoV-229E and NL63 while beta coronaviruses include OC43 and HKU1 [9]. The binary human viruses (HCoV-229E and HCoV-NL63) that are identified as the alpha coronavirus can infect animals and cause severe illness. The amino peptidase N (APN) protein is present in the host and acts as a receptor for HCoV-229E [10]. The Type II transmembrane protein CD13 is termed an APN protein that originates on the respiratory and intestinal epithelial cells. The APNs are Zn^{2+}dependent proteases and they have the capability to break down the protein of N terminal neutral amino acids. Furthermore, the beta SARS-CoV is able to bind to the carbohydrates that are presented in a galectin fold-like structure found in the S1 NTD. The SARS-CoV was first discovered in 2002 and the (ACE-2) receptor was responsible for the virus [11]. Type I main membrane protein is a mono-carboxypeptidase that hydrolyzes angiotensin II and it is found in a substantial fraction of ACE2 receptors expressed in lung tissue. When a coronavirus infects the host, the calcium-dependent (C-type) lectins are predicted. Humans, mammals and birds are all afflicted by the coronavirus infection in humans as it affects the respiratory tract, the gastrointestinal tract, the hepatic system and the nervous system. Acute and persistent infections are both possible [12]. The α, β, γ, and δ are four different types of coronaviruses in which the alpha and beta are responsible for infections. Acute lung injury is caused by H5N1, SARS-CoV and H1N1 while acute respiratory distress syndrome (ARDS) could cause failure and death of the pulmonary region. The following are two possibilities that are likely to explain the creation of novel coronaviruses: a) natural selection in an animal host prior to and after zoonotic transmission and b) natural selection in humans after zoonotic transmission. Clinical types and risk factors are highly variable, resulting in scientific data ranging from asymptomatic to lethal. The basic symptoms of coronavirus include: cough, sore throat, breathlessness, fever, and the patient must be quarantined for 2-14 days after infection. Following the (H1N1), 1957 (H2N2), 1968 (H3N2) and 2009 Pandemic flu (H1N1), the WHO had declared a new coronavirus outbreak pandemic on March 11, 2020 [13] (Fig. **1**).

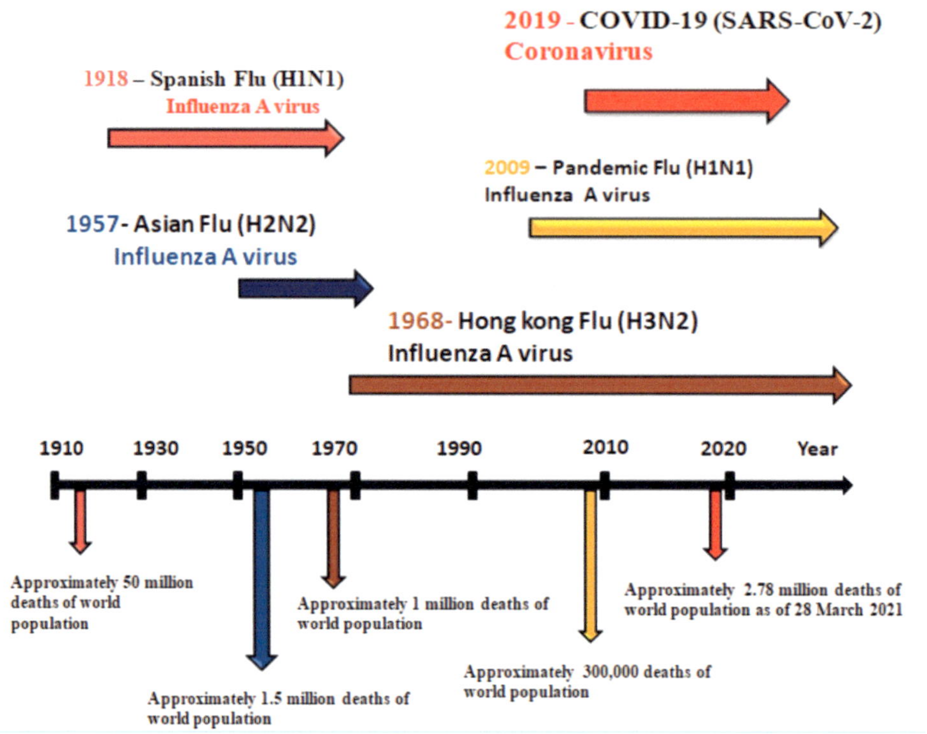

Fig. (1). A timeline of the five pandemics that have occurred since 1918 as well as the viruses that have remained circulating globally ever since.

2. HISTORICAL BACKGROUND, ORIGIN AND THE TRANSMISSION OF CORONAVIRUS

Coronavirus (CoV) was first discovered in the 1960s. The International Committee on the Taxonomy of the Coronavirus study group utilised relative genomics to evaluate and screen the replicative proteins in open reading frames as well as to differentiate and identify CoV at different cluster ranks [14]. CoV is linked with varying degrees of illness. In the past, SARS (in 2002–2003) and (MERS) (in 2012) had resulted to large scale pandemics. In the 1960s, the coronavirus was often found in animals and birds especially camels, rats, and bats [15] (Fig. **2**). The taxonomy of coronavirus is as follows: genus -Coronavirus, family Coronaviridae, and order Nidovirales [16]. From 2002 to 2003, a similar virus was identified which had infected humans and it was discovered to be the cause of SARS. The COVID-19 infection is triggered by a virus containing a positive-sense RNA genome of 30 kb. The coronaviruses found in *Manis javanica* and *Rhinolophus sinicus*are said to have approximately 74% to 95% similarity with this virus [17]. A major source of coronavirus was found to be off the bat, out of which, a few of them had infected humans. Based on the current studies, the SARS and MERS viruses which were first discovered in 2002 and 2012, were transmitted zoonotically by bats that had used palm civets and camels as intermediate hosts. According to the latest studies, SARS-CoV-2 is a bat-adapted coronavirus that has transferred to humans *via* zoonotic transmission. The Malayan pangolin coronavirus has been determined to be 99% identical to a new coronavirus. The pangolin-CoV receptor-binding domain (RBD) differs from SARS-CoV-2 by only one amino acid; pangolins infected with COVID-19 have shown pathological symptoms which are similar to humans and their blood circulating antibodies are able to react with the SARS-CoV-2 spike protein [18].

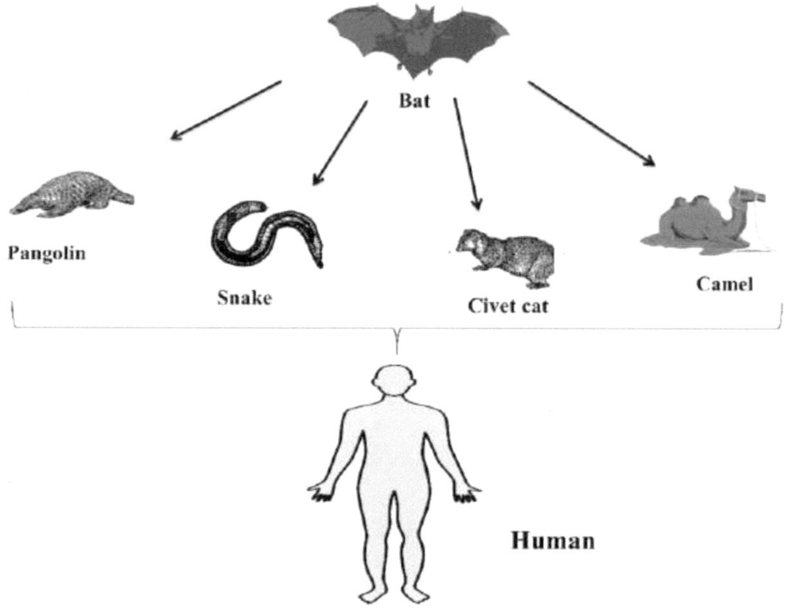

Fig. (2). Different viruses found in different mammals such as SARS virus in civet cat, MERS virus in camel and SARS-CoV-2 in pangolin or snake.

3. CLASSIFICATION OF CORONAVIRUS

Coronaviruses are viruses that belong to the Coronaviridae family which is the most important family in the Nidovirales order. The coronaviridae family is divided into two subfamilies: torovirinae and orthocoronavirinae, each of which consists of four genera: α, β, γ, and *δ* coronavirus [19]. CoVs are commonly found in humans and birds, but they can also be discovered in other animals (Fig. **3**). Alpha and beta coronaviruses are found in mammals whereas birds and mammalian species would be infected through gamma coronavirus. Delta coronaviruses on the other hand would infect both birds and mammals. Animal CoV poses a substantial threat to livestock and it is suspected to be the cause of financial losses in domestic animals and birds. Moreover, animals can infect humans and spread infection through human-to-human transmission, which is uncommon [20].

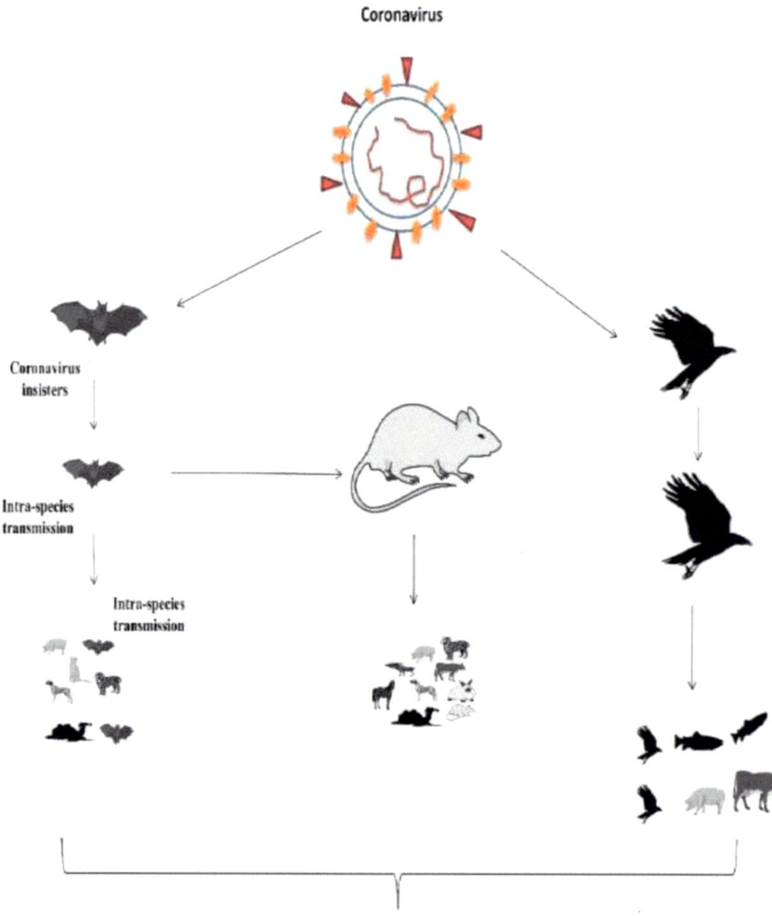

(Fig. 3) contd.....

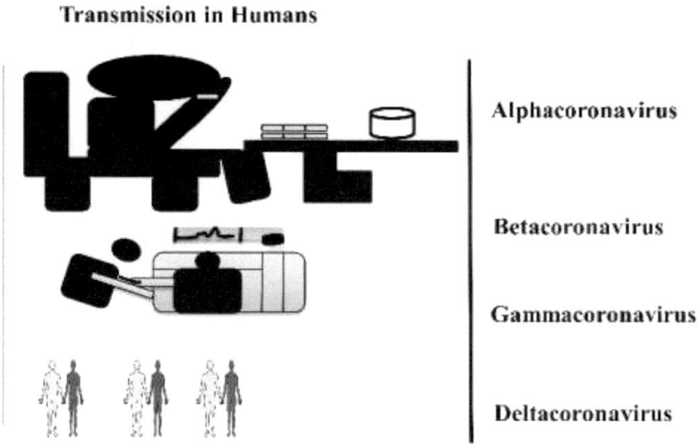

Fig.(3). Animal to human transmission of a virus is a rich source of ingestion of infected animals as well as coming into close contact with an infected person and the virus can be transmitted to a healthy individual.

3.1. Differences and Similarities Between SARS, MERS, and the nCoV-2019

3.1.1. Similarities and Differences

SARS-CoV was discovered in 2002 to 2003 and it was referred to as a Severe Acute Respiratory Syndrome. It occurred in Guandong Province, China with a total of 8098 cases identified and a death rate of 774 [21]. Coughing, shortness of breath, fever as well as other serious complications such as pneumonia and kidney failure were the symptoms of SARS-CoV. The incubation period would last from two to fourteen days. According to research, SARS-like CoVs were found in civets and raccoon dogs from the local Chinese markets. SARS-CoV was first detected in bats and small animals before it was transmitted to humans. Several SARS-CoVs have been identified in bats from various regions of China through research. Various studies have revealed that the ACE-2 receptors have an SARS binding affinity [22]. The SARS-CoV consists of the S protein, which has the highest binding affinity towards the ACE-2 receptor, which is found in human lungs and would eventually affect the airway epithelial. In 2012, **MERS-CoV** was identified in Saudi Arabia. The symptoms and incubation period of MERS-CoV were found to be similar to SARS-CoV [23]. MERS-CoV was detected in 27 countries, with an estimated total of 2506 cases and a death rate of 862. MERS-related CoVs (MERS-CoVs) were discovered in bats, suggesting that the dromedary camels had transmitted the MERS-CoV to humans. According to studies conducted, the camel MERS-CoV strain was known as the human MERS-CoV strain. MERS-CoV, like SARS-CoV, consists of S proteins that are harmful to humans [24]. MERS-CoV had a strong affinity for human DPP4, infected human cells and triggered the outbreak in 2012 [25]. As previously described, nCoV-2019 was discovered in Wuhan, China, and was later given the name of COVID-19. SARS-CoV-2, the third human CoV, would induce respiratory failure and had a similar incubation time to SARS-CoV and MERS-CoV infections [26]. Cases in China and around the world are on the rise since December 2019. Based on the patients' samples, the nCoV-19 virus has been identified as a beta coronavirus. According to the findings of the study, SARS-CoV-2 is a new virus that is similar to SARS-CoV and MERS-CoV, in which both were found in bats [27]. The SARS-CoV-2 virus contains several proteins, one of which is known as the spike protein. The spike protein has the highest binding affinity for the ACE-2 receptor which would cause damage to the lungs' epithelial cells (Table **1**).

Table 1. Classification of human coronavirus.

Classification of Human Coronavirus								References
Strain	HcoV-229E	HcoV-OC43	SARS-CoV	HcoV-NL63	HcoV-HKU1	MERS-CoV	SARS-CoV-2	[28-34]
Discovery	1966	1967	2003	2004	2005	2012	2019	[35-40]
Genera-Lineage	α	β-A	β-B	α	β-A	β-C	β-B	[41-47]
Cellular Receptor	AminopeptidaseN (CD13)	9-*O*-Acetylatedsialic acid(SA)	ACE2	ACE2	9-*O*-Acetylatedsialic acid(SA)	DPP4	ACE2	[48-53]
Natural Host	Bats	Rodents	Bats	Bats	Rodents	Bats	Bats	[54-60]
Breathing Symptom	gentle	gentle	Severe	gentle	gentle	Severe	Severe	

4. STRUCTURE OF CORONAVIRUS AND ROLE OF THEIR PROTEINS

4.1. Coronavirus Structure

The SARS-CoV-2 virus has a spherical shape and it is composed of positive RNA viruses consisting of a single strand which comprises spike proteins on the surface of the virus. The coronavirus is a spherical virus with a crown-like structure [61]. The word corona means "crown" in Latin as the virus appears as a royal crown under an electron microscope. The coronavirus is encased in a lipid bilayer and consists of several proteins including S, E, M, and N [62] (Fig. **4**).The proteins are situated on the surface of the virus; however, in the viral RNA, the N protein shows interaction with RNA and it is found in the viral particle's core, where it forms the nucleocapsid. The S protein is known as the leading protein due to its high binding affinity for the ACE-2 receptor, which is found in the human lungs [63]. The spike protein has two parts S1 and S2 which are produced by the breakdown of the S protein through the host furin-like proteases. These spike proteins are present on the viral particle. When compared to the other proteins in the viral particle, the M protein is discovered in large amounts whereas the E protein is found in extremely small amounts [64]. M protein provides the virus its shape and works with E protein to orchestrate virus assembly and the creation of mature viral envelopes, therefore, could explain the difference in abundance. E protein also assists in the release of viral particles from the host cells, among other things. During viral assembly, the N protein would bind viral RNA as it is necessary for viral RNA packaging into the viral particle [65].

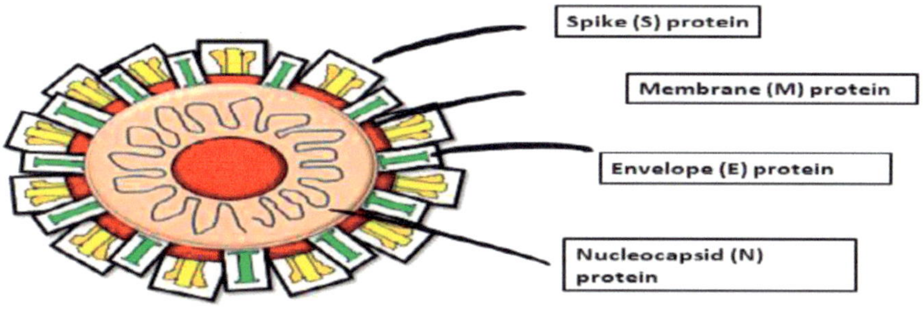

Fig. (4). Structure of coronavirus.

4.2. Spike Protein and its Drawbacks into the Host Body

The novel coronavirus can be transmitted through respiratory droplets, produced by coughing and sneezing. CoVs, the enveloped positive-stranded RNA virus family, are classified into three major genera or groups: α-CoVs (group 1), β-CoVs (group 2) and γ-CoVs (group 3) [66]. Based on the structure of SARS-Co--2, they are made up of four proteins: S, E, M and N that encapsulate a single-stranded viral RNA. The spike tends to interact with the host cell receptors. The host cell protease divides the spike protein into S1 and S2, one of which is a transmembrane protease serine 2 (TMPRSS2) [67]. The S1 subunit's primary function is to attach to harmless receptors on the host cell, whereas the S2 subunits would facilitate the membrane fusion Fig.(**5**). Therefore, it is most likely that the first approach is to develop a vaccine, followed by developing monoclonal antibodies that would attach with the spike protein and inhibit human cell interaction. Another potential target is the transmembrane protease serine two, which is required for coronavirus entry and viral spread. According to recent protein studies, the SARS-CoV-2 has a strong binding affinity to the human Angiotensin Converting-Enzyme 2 (ACE-2) receptors, which may be used as a mechanism for SARS entry [68] (Fig. **6**). Type 2 alveolar cells which are found in the respiratory tract, have a high expression of ACE-2 receptors. ACE-2 receptors on the other hand, are found in a wide range of extrapulmonary tissues, including the heart, kidney, endothelium, and intestine. As a result, the interaction sites between ACE-2 and the spike protein should be considered as a potential drug target. A natural flavonoid called Hesperidin has already been identified in recent computational studies as a compound that is expected to bind with the binding interface of the spike ACE-2 complex [69]. According to the studies, spike proteins have the highest binding with the ACE-2 receptor, which could lead to severe lung injury.

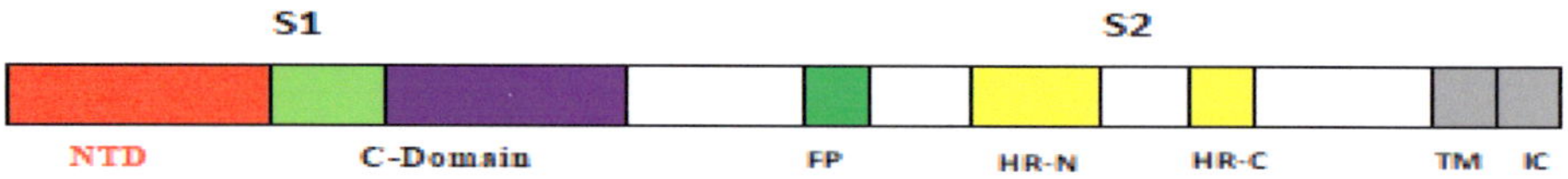

Sequence similarity in S1	Alpha-CoV NL63	Alpha-CoV TGEV	Beta-CoV MHV	Beta-CoV BCoV	Beta-CoV SARS	Gama-CoV IBV	Control (SARS pol)
Alpha-CoV NL63	100	31	10	11	10	17	7
Alpha-CoV TGEV		100	10	10	9	9	6
Beta-CoV MHV			100	58	22	10	9
Beta-CoV BCoV				100	21	11	7
Beta-CoV SARS					100	8	4
Gama-CoV IBV						100	6
Control (SARS pol)							Average +3*SD =11

Fig. (5). Three coronavirus genera or groups' spike proteins.

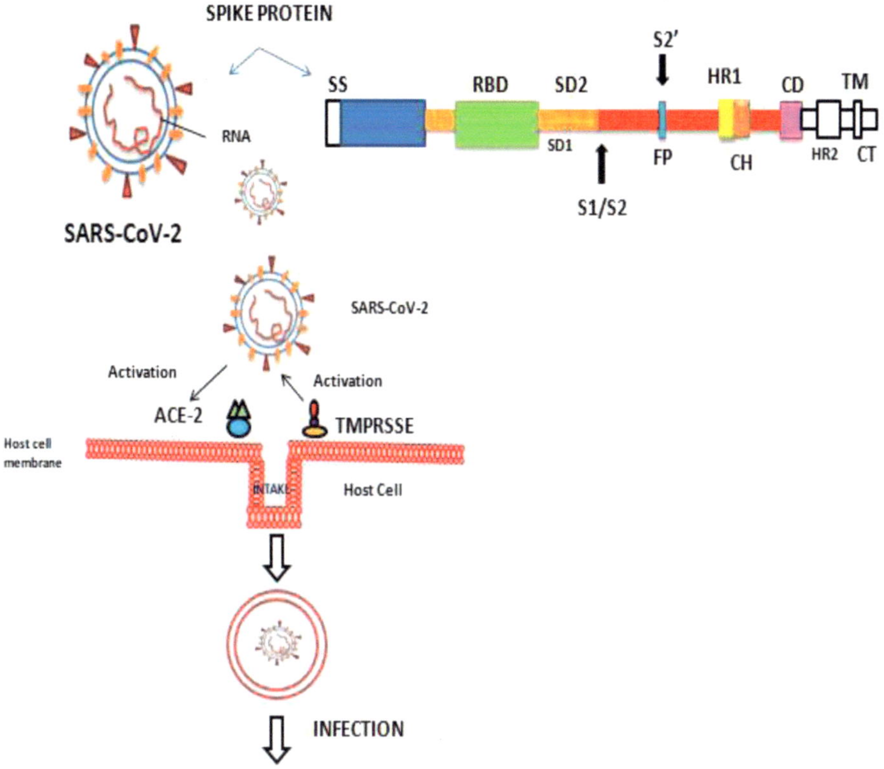

Fig. (6). The coronavirus has several types of proteins on its surfaces, including S, E, M, N, as well as the spike protein, which is the leading protein of the coronavirus which would bind with the host cell receptor. The spike protein is chopped into two domains, S1 and S2, and one other protein is the transmembrane protease serine 2 (TMPRSS2). The presence of ACE-2 receptors in type 2 alveolar cells can be found in the respiratory tract. As a result of the study, it is clear that the coronavirus binds to the ACE-2 and the ACE-2 down-regulates the receptor, contributing to severe lung injury.

5. MECHANISM OF VIRAL ENTRY

The coronavirus is a huge class of viruses; it is not one specific illness; they are giant enveloped RNA viruses with a large RNA genome that can cause the (SARS) syndrome [70]. The coronavirus diagram depicts the viral entry and their involvement in various steps to damage the host cell. The host cell plasma membrane contains one protein receptor called CEACAM-1 which is responsible for the entry of novel coronavirus inside the host body (Fig. **7**). With the spike proteins around the virus, they would bind to the CEACAM-1 and facilitate the receptor-mediated endocytosis, which would attract the virus to the host cell *via* conformational changes and adaptation in the plasma membrane [71]. Once the uncoating occurs, these proteins would move and the content of the virus is released into the genomic RNA host cell cytoplasm. This genomic RNA is known as a genomic RNA positive and it is nearly 30,000 nucleotides long. Then, the host cell machinery namely ribosomes would translate this genomic strand into two polyproteins, which are also known as polyprotein1a and polyprotein1b [72]. Consequently, numerous non-structural proteins would be obtained from the breakdown of the polyprotein which includes the RNA-dependent RNA polymerase (RdRp), helicases and non-structural proteins (nsp3, nsp4, nsp6) [73]. It has been stated that the non-structural protein would initiate the multiplication of the coronavirus. The replication of the coronavirus takes place in the endoplasmic reticulum membrane conscription to form double-membrane vesicles that are known as DMV. The RdRp and helicase which are localized within the DMV drive the production of sub-genomic RNA [74]. The entire sense RNA would undergo two events. Firstly, it can replicate back into sense RNA, which is exactly the same scenario during uncoating in the original virus. Secondly, a complete sense RNA can be transcribed by using a method known as discontinuous transcription in which a complete sense RNA can be produced. Furthermore, it could transcribe a slew of different RNA, all of which are truly mRNA that should be translated into different proteins, thus resulting in the formation of N copies of proteins from a single RNA. After synthesis, transmembrane structural proteins S, M, and E are inserted and folded inside the E.R before they are transported into the Golgi (ERGIC) compartment [75]. To form a nucleocapsid, the N proteins would bind to the viral genomic RNA inside the cytoplasm. Once the final virion gathering occurs in the intermediate compartment that is known as ERGIC, the mature virion is exocytosed into the smooth-walled vesicles and releases the viral progeny which matures the coronavirus to infect other cells [76].

6. MODES OF TRANSMISSION

The transmission of novel coronavirus is preferably administered *via* normal routes which include a close contact with the infected person as well as direct transmission and airborne. Some of the common modes of transmission include sneezing and coughing, continuous acts of touching the face, nose and eyes (Fig. **8**). Viral shedding occurs from the respiratory tract, saliva, feces and urine, resulting in the spread of the virus to other locations. The viral load is greater and lasts longer in patients with severe COVID-19. COVID-19 also has been reported to spread from infected patients to health care workers and flight attendants who were in close contact with them [77].

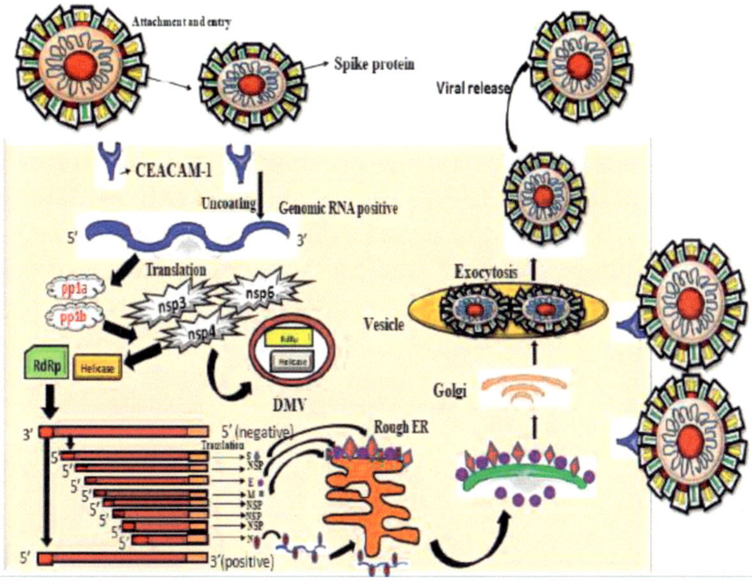

Fig. (7). The mechanism of coronavirus is depicted in the diagram; the coronavirus contains various types of proteins, the leading protein is known as the spike protein; the spike protein enters the host body and attaches to the CEACAM-1 present in the host cell, and through conformational changes, receptor-mediated endocytosis would occur and the virus is released towards the genomic RNA and translate this genomic strand into two polyproteins and many non-structural proteins. Non-structural proteins such as RdRp and helicase are localized into the DMV and drive the production of sub-genomic RNA from which structural and accessory proteins are produced in the next phase of translation. Then, from one RNA N copies of proteins form, the transmembrane structural proteins would enter the ER and are transported into the Golgi compartment and the mammalian cell nucleus.

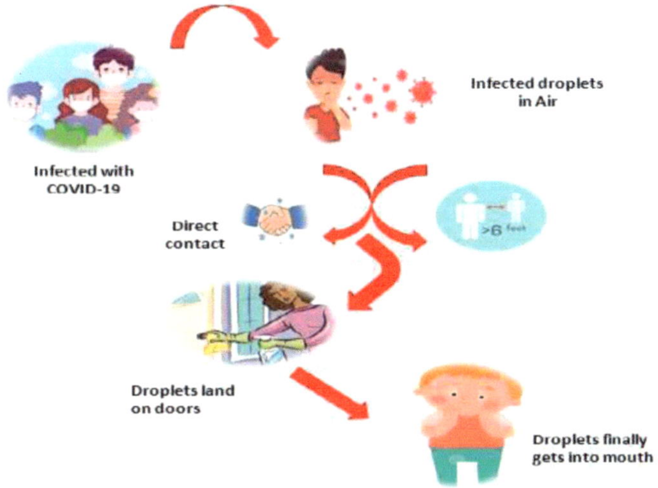

Fig. (8). Modes of transmission of COVID-19.

7. TREATMENTS OF COVID-19

A large number of populations around the world have suffered from novel coronavirus. As such, various pieces of evidence have suggested that there is a lack of concrete proof for effective antiviral treatments for COVID-19 [78]. In the diagnosis and treatment of COVID-19 pneumonia, currently available treatments are primarily focused on symptomatic and respiratory support. The treatment of coronavirus can be done through antiviral agents, natural products, and vaccination [79] (Fig. **9**).

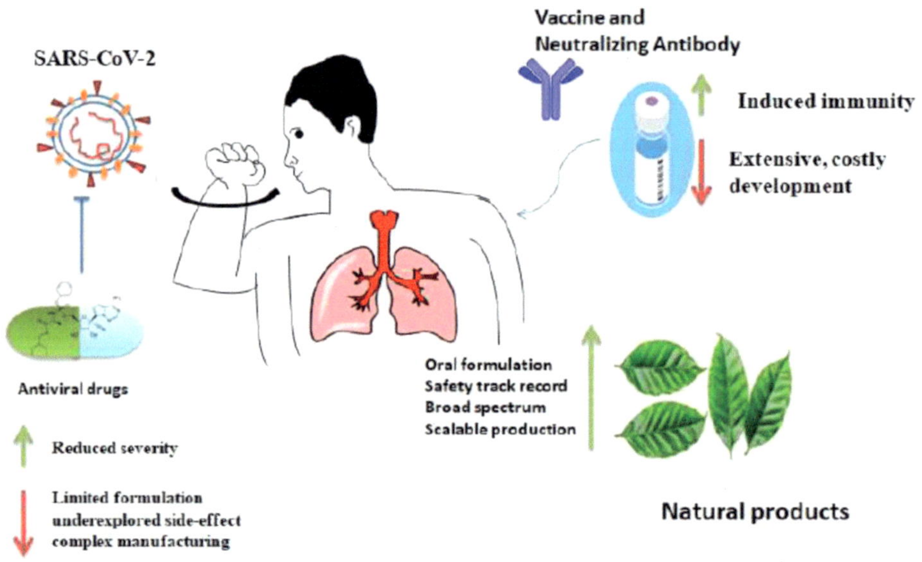

Fig. (9). Current prevention of COVID-19.

7.1. Antiviral Agents

There are various clinical manifestations of the novel coronavirus that occur through replication. A variety of researches are still ongoing to discover the most effective antiviral treatments of nCoV. For coronavirus therapy, antiviral therapies are being investigated. These drugs would suppress the ACE2 and TMPRSS2 receptors to inhibit the entry of the virus as the viral replication could be particularly active during the early stages of COVID-19. Despite the urgent need for randomised controlled trials to find the most appropriate COVID-19 antiviral therapy, several agents are currently utilised globally [80]. Table **2** highlights the most commonly used agents and their mechanisms of action.

Table 2. Antivirals drugs for the management of COVID-19

Antivirals Drugs For The Management of COVID-19					References
Group	Inhibitors of viral RNA polymerase/RNA synthesis	Inhibitors of viral protein synthesis	Viral entry inhibitors	Immunomodulators	[81-84]
Drugs	Remdesivir	Lopinavir/ritonavir	Hydroxychloroquine	Nitazoxanide	
	Favipiravir		Chloroquine	Ivermectin	
Mechanism of Action	**Remdesivir** (Adenosine nucleotide analog, RdRp inhibitors)	Protease inhibitor	Increasing endosomal pH, which is required for cell fusion, and interfere with ACE-2 receptor	**Nitazoxanide** (Interference with viral replication-related host-regulated pathways)	[85-90]
	Favipiravir (Guanosinenucleotide analog, RdRp inhibitor)			**Ivermectin** (Importin 1 heterodimer inhibition of nuclear import of host and viral proteins)	
Dosing	**Remdesivir** (Day 1: 200mg, IV Day 2-5 (or 10): 100mg/day, IV	Day 1 to 10 or (14): 400mg/ 100mg x 2/day, orally	Day 1 to 5: 2 X 200 mg/day, orally	-	[91-95]
	Favipiravir (Day 1: 2X1600mg, Day 2 to 7 (or 10): 2 X 600mg/day		Day 1 to 5 (or 10): 2 X 500mg/day, orally	-	

7.2. Natural Products

Treatment of coronavirus through natural products which have effective antiviral activity towards human CoVs, plays a key role in the development of new antiviral prophylactics. Herbal compounds which are comprised of phytoconstituents with effective antiviral, anti-inflammatory and antimicrobial properties, such as Dihydrotanshinone, Griffithsin, Emodin, Tannic acid, Gallic acid and Withanone are recent trends in the community. These phytoconstituents are believed to possess the ability to adapt the immune response therefore, could be beneficial for the treatment against COVID-19 [96]. The lists of herbal agents which are effective against coronavirus are shown in (Table **3**).

Table 3. Natural products potentially effective for COVID-19

Natural Products Potentially Effective for COVID-19							References
Herbal Agents	Dihydrotanshinone	Griffithsin	Emodin	Tannic acid	Gallic acid	Withanone	[97-102]
Virus Inhibited	MERS-CoV	MERS-CoV	SARS-CoV	SARS-CoV	SARS-CoV-2	SARS-CoV-2	
Drug Targets	S protein of MERS-CoV	S protein of MERS-CoV	S protein and ACE2 interaction	3CLPro	RdRp	TMPRSS2	[103-107]
Mechanism of Action	Block MERS-CoV entry using pre- and post-attachment assay	Inhibit spike protein function during entry	Blocked the binding of S protein to ACE2 using biotinylated ELISA assay, IC50: 200 mM	Inhibition of 3CLPro, IC50: 3 μM	High binding affinity to RdRp tested by molecular docking	Bind and interact at the catalytic site of TMPRSS2	

7.3. Vaccines

Currently, COVID-19 vaccination could be the only definitive and preventive treatment option to fight the virus. Due to this, there are several vaccines under clinical trials. In addition to antiviral agents, widespread use of the COVID-19 vaccine is a promising strategy to bring an end to the current pandemic. Dozens of COVID-19 vaccines which are developed by various organizations are in various stages of clinical testing [108]. The list of vaccines under clinical trials is shown in Fig. (**10**).

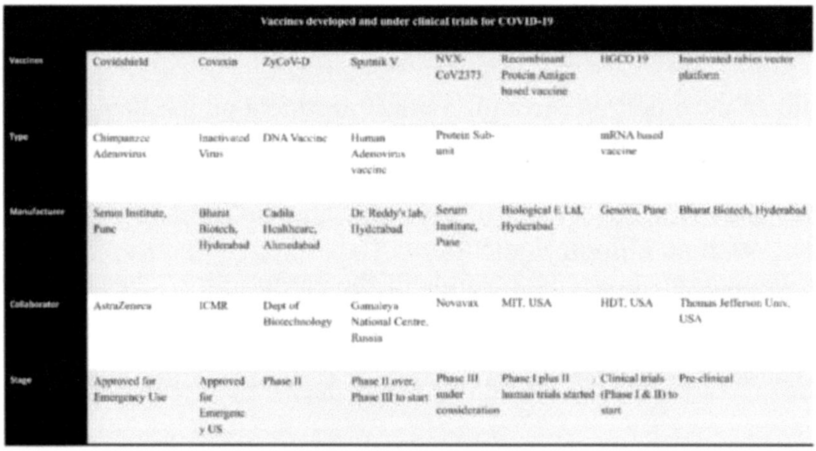

Vaccines developed and under clinical trials for COVID-19								
Vaccines	Covidshield	Covaxin	ZyCoV-D	Sputnik V	NVX-CoV2373	Recombinant Protein Antigen based vaccine	HGCO 19	Inactivated rabies vector platform
Type	Chimpanzee Adenovirus	Inactivated Virus	DNA Vaccine	Human Adenovirus vaccine	Protein Sub-unit		mRNA based vaccine	
Manufacturer	Serum Institute, Pune	Bharat Biotech, Hyderabad	Cadila Healthcare, Ahmedabad	Dr. Reddy's lab, Hyderabad	Serum Institute, Pune	Biological E Ltd, Hyderabad	Genova, Pune	Bharat Biotech, Hyderabad
Collaborator	AstraZeneca	ICMR	Dept of Biotechnology	Gamaleya National Centre, Russia	Novavax	MIT, USA	HDT, USA	Thomas Jefferson Univ, USA
Stage	Approved for Emergency Use	Approved for Emergenc y US	Phase II	Phase II over, Phase III to start	Phase III under consideration	Phase I plus II human trials started	Clinical trials (Phase I & II) to start	Pre-clinical

Fig. (10). Vaccines developed and under clinical trials for COVID-19.

CONCLUSION

COVID-19, a virus that is still persistent even today has infected a large number of populations around the world for the past couple of years, just like its predecessors SARS-CoV and MERS-CoV. Coronavirus is encased in a lipid bilayer and consists of several proteins including S, E, M and N. Spike protein would damage lung cells after binding with ACE-2 receptors. The S1 domain is responsible for receptor recognition as it would bind to the host cell receptor, while the S2 domain is responsible for fusion. Moreover, coronaviruses are divided into four genera such as α, β, γ and δ. Thus, the current report has dwelled on the pathogen's characteristics, modes of transmission and the origin of coronavirus to provide conceptual information on various treatment approaches for COVID-19.

CONSENT FOR PUBLICATION

Not applicable.

CONFLICT OF INTEREST

The author declares no conflict of interest, financial or otherwise.

ACKNOWLEDGEMENTS

Declared none.

REFERENCES

[1] Kotfis k, Roberson SW, Wilson JE, Dabrowski W, Pun BT, Ely EW. COVID-19 : ICU delirium management during SARS-CoV-2 pandemic. Crit Care 2020; 176: 1-9.

[2] Kochi AN, Tagliari AP, Forleo GB, Fassini GM, Tondo C. Cardiac and arrhythmic complications in patients with COVID-19. J Cardiovasc Electrophysiol 2020; 31(5): 1003-8. [http://dx.doi.org/10.1111/jce.14479] [PMID: 32270559]

[3] Adhikari N, Amin SA, Jha T. Dissecting the drug development strategies against sars-cov-2 through diverse computational modeling techniques. Methods Pharmacol Toxicol. 2020; 1-104.

[4] Sahoo S, Rakshit R. Novel human coronavirus sars-cov-2 and Covid-19: a brief review. Int J Pharma Bio Sci 2021; 11(1): 273-83. [http://dx.doi.org/10.22376/ijpbs/lpr.2021.11.1.L273-283]

[5] Liang Y, Wang ML, Chien CS, *et al.* Highlight of immune pathogenic response and hematopathologic effect in sars-cov, mers-cov, and sars-cov-2 infection. Front Immunol 2020; 11: 1022. [http://dx.doi.org/10.3389/fimmu.2020.01022] [PMID: 32574260]

[6] Huang Y, Yang C, Xu X, Xu W, Liu S. Structural and functional properties of SARS-CoV-2 spike protein: potential antivirus drug development for COVID-19. Acta Pharmacol Sin 2020; 41(9): 1141-9. [http://dx.doi.org/10.1038/s41401-020-0485-4] [PMID: 32747721]

[7] Satarker S, Nampoothiri M. Structural proteins in severe acute respiratory syndrome coronavirus-2. Arch Med Res 2020; 51(6): 482-91.

[http://dx.doi.org/10.1016/j.arcmed.2020.05.012] [PMID: 32493627]

[8] Belouzard S, Millet JK, Licitra BN, Whittaker GR. Mechanisms of coronavirus cell entry mediated by the viral spike protein. Viruses 2012; 4(6): 1011-33. [http://dx.doi.org/10.3390/v4061011] [PMID: 22816037]

[9] Xiu L, Zhang C, Wu Z, Peng J. Establishment and application of a universal coronavirus screening method using MALDI-TOF mass spectrometry. Front Microbiol 2017; 8: 1510. [http://dx.doi.org/10.3389/fmicb.2017.01510] [PMID: 28848521]

[10] Lau SKP, Woo PCY, Li KSM, *et al.* Discovery of a novel coronavirus, China Rattus coronavirus HKU24, from Norway rats supports the murine origin of Betacoronavirus 1 and has implications for the ancestor of Betacoronavirus lineage A. J Virol 2015; 89(6): 3076-92. [http://dx.doi.org/10.1128/JVI.02420-14] [PMID: 25552712]

[11] Lee C, Choi WJ. Overview of COVID-19 inflammatory pathogenesis from the therapeutic perspective. Arch Pharm Res 2021; 44(1): 99-116. [http://dx.doi.org/10.1007/s12272-020-01301-7] [PMID: 33398692]

[12] Liu L, Wei Q, Lin Q, *et al.* Anti–spike IgG causes severe acute lung injury by skewing macrophage responses during acute SARS-CoV infection. JCI Insight 2019; 4(4): e123158. [http://dx.doi.org/10.1172/jci.insight.123158] [PMID: 30830861]

[13] Hsu LY, Chia PY, Lim JFY. The novel coronavirus (sars-cov-2) epidemic. Ann Acad Med Singap 2020; 49(3): 105-7. [http://dx.doi.org/10.47102/annals-acadmedsg.202051] [PMID: 32200398]

[14] V'kovski P, Kratzel A, Steiner S, Stalder H, Thiel V. Coronavirus biology and replication: implications for SARS-CoV-2. Nat Rev Microbiol 2021; 19(3): 155-70. [http://dx.doi.org/10.1038/s41579-020-00468-6] [PMID: 33116300]

[15] Al-Salihi KA, Khalaf JM. The emerging SARS-CoV, MERS-CoV, and SARS-CoV-2: An insight into the viruses zoonotic aspects. Vet World 2021; 14(1): 190-9. [http://dx.doi.org/10.14202/vetworld.2021.190-199] [PMID: 33642804]

[16] Goldsmith CS, Tatti KM, Ksiazek TG, *et al.* Ultrastructural characterization of SARS coronavirus. Emerg Infect Dis 2004; 10(2): 320-6. [http://dx.doi.org/10.3201/eid1002.030913] [PMID: 15030705]

[17] Nadeem MS, Zamzami MA, Choudhry H, *et al.* Origin, potential therapeutic targets and treatment for coronavirus disease (covid-19). Pathogens 2020; 9(4): 307. [http://dx.doi.org/10.3390/pathogens9040307] [PMID: 32331255]

[18] Xiao K, Zhai J, Feng Y, *et al.* Isolation of SARS-CoV-2-related coronavirus from Malayan pangolins. Nature 2020; 583(7815): 286-9. [http://dx.doi.org/10.1038/s41586-020-2313-x] [PMID: 32380510]

[19] Weiss SR, Navas-Martin S. Coronavirus pathogenesis and the emerging pathogen severe acute respiratory syndrome coronavirus. Microbiol Mol Biol Rev 2005; 69(4): 635-64. [http://dx.doi.org/10.1128/MMBR.69.4.635-664.2005] [PMID: 16339739]

[20] Miłek J, Blicharz-Domańska K. Coronaviruses in avian species – review with focus on epidemiology and diagnosis in wild birds. J Vet Res (Pulawy) 2018; 62(3): 249-55. [http://dx.doi.org/10.2478/jvetres-2018-0035] [PMID: 30584600]

[21] Park SE. Epidemiology, virology, and clinical features of severe acute respiratory syndrome - coronavirus-2 (SARS-CoV-2; Coronavirus Disease-19). Clinical and Experimental Pediatrics 2020; 63(4): 119-24. [http://dx.doi.org/10.3345/cep.2020.00493] [PMID: 32252141]

[22] Ashour HM, Elkhatib WF, Rahman MM, Elshabrawy HA. Insights into the recent 2019 novel coronavirus (sars-cov-2) in light of past human coronavirus outbreaks. Pathogens 2020; 9(3): 186. [http://dx.doi.org/10.3390/pathogens9030186] [PMID: 32143502]

[23] Assiri A, McGeer A, Perl TM, *et al.* Hospital outbreak of Middle East respiratory syndrome coronavirus. N Engl J Med 2013; 369(5): 407-16.
[http://dx.doi.org/10.1056/NEJMoa1306742] [PMID: 23782161]

[24] Lu G, Wang Q, Gao GF. Bat-to-human: spike features determining 'host jump' of coronaviruses SARS-CoV, MERS-CoV, and beyond. Trends Microbiol 2015; 23(8): 468-78.
[http://dx.doi.org/10.1016/j.tim.2015.06.003] [PMID: 26206723]

[25] Li Y, Zhang Z, Yang L, *et al.* The mers-cov receptor dpp4 as a candidate binding target of the sars-cov-2 spike. iScience 2020; 23(6): 101160.
[http://dx.doi.org/10.1016/j.isci.2020.101160] [PMID: 32405622]

[26] Xu J, Zhao S, Teng T, *et al.* Systematic comparison of two animal-to-human transmitted human coronaviruses: SARS-CoV-2 and SARS-CoV. Viruses 2020; 12(2): 244.
[http://dx.doi.org/10.3390/v12020244] [PMID: 32098422]

[27] Giri R, Bhardwaj T, Shegane M, *et al.* Understanding COVID-19 *via* comparative analysis of dark proteomes of SARS-CoV-2, human SARS and bat SARS-like coronaviruses. Cell Mol Life Sci 2021; 78(4): 1655-88.
[http://dx.doi.org/10.1007/s00018-020-03603-x] [PMID: 32712910]

[28] Bonavia A, Zelus BD, Wentworth DE, Talbot PJ, Holmes KV. Identification of a receptor-binding domain of the spike glycoprotein of human coronavirus HCoV-229E. J Virol 2003; 77(4): 2530-8.
[http://dx.doi.org/10.1128/JVI.77.4.2530-2538.2003] [PMID: 12551991]

[29] Zhang S, Tuo J, Huang X, *et al.* Epidemiology characteristics of human coronaviruses in patients with respiratory infection symptoms and phylogenetic analysis of HCoV-OC43 during 2010-2015 in Guangzhou. PLoS One 2018; 13(1): e0191789.
[http://dx.doi.org/10.1371/journal.pone.0191789] [PMID: 29377913]

[30] Hasöksüz M, Kiliç S, Saraç F. Coronaviruses and SARS-COV-2. Turk J Med Sci 2020; 50(SI-1): 549-56.
[http://dx.doi.org/10.3906/sag-2004-127] [PMID: 32293832]

[31] Abdul-Rasool S, Fielding BC. Understanding human coronavirus HCoV-NL63. Open Virol J 2010; 4(1): 76-84.
[http://dx.doi.org/10.2174/1874357901004010076] [PMID: 20700397]

[32] Zhao Q, Li S, Xue F, *et al.* Structure of the main protease from a global infectious human coronavirus, HCoV-HKU1. J Virol 2008; 82(17): 8647-55.
[http://dx.doi.org/10.1128/JVI.00298-08] [PMID: 18562531]

[33] Oboho IK, Tomczyk SM, Al-Asmari AM, *et al.* 2014 MERS-CoV outbreak in Jeddah--a link to health care facilities. N Engl J Med 2015; 372(9): 846-54.
[http://dx.doi.org/10.1056/NEJMoa1408636] [PMID: 25714162]

[34] Kim D, Lee JY, Yang JS, Kim JW, Kim VN, Chang H. The architecture of SARS-CoV-2 transcriptome. Cell 2020; 181(4): 914-921.e10.
[http://dx.doi.org/10.1016/j.cell.2020.04.011] [PMID: 32330414]

[35] Shirato K, Kanou K, Kawase M, Matsuyama S. Clinical isolates of human coronavirus 229E bypass the endosome for cell entry. J Virol 2016; 91(1): e01387-16.
[PMID: 27733646]

[36] Szczepanski A, Owczarek K, Bzowska M, *et al.* Canine respiratory coronavirus, bovine coronavirus, and human coronavirus OC43: receptors and attachment factors. Viruses 2019; 11(4): 328.
[http://dx.doi.org/10.3390/v11040328] [PMID: 30959796]

[37] Naddeo V, Liu H. Editorial Perspectives: 2019 novel coronavirus (SARS-CoV-2): what is its fate in urban water cycle and how can the water research community respond? Environ Sci Water Res Technol 2020; 6(5): 1213-6.
[http://dx.doi.org/10.1039/D0EW90015J]

[38] Esper F, Weibel C, Ferguson D, Landry ML, Kahn JS. Coronavirus HKU1 Infection in the United States. Emerg Infect Dis 2006; 12(5): 775-9. [http://dx.doi.org/10.3201/eid1205.051316] [PMID: 16704837]

[39] Ba Abduallah MM, Hemida MG. Comparative analysis of the genome structure and organization of the Middle East respiratory syndrome coronavirus (MERS-COV) 2012 to 2019 revealing evidence for virus strain barcoding, zoonotic transmission, and selection pressure. Rev Med Virol 2021; 31(1): 1-12. [http://dx.doi.org/10.1002/rmv.2150] [PMID: 32803835]

[40] Yan Y, Chang L, Wang L. Laboratory testing of SARS-CoV, MERS-CoV, and SARS-CoV-2 (2019-nCoV): Current status, challenges, and countermeasures. Rev Med Virol 2020; 30(3): e2106. [http://dx.doi.org/10.1002/rmv.2106] [PMID: 32302058]

[41] Kuri T, Eriksson KK, Putics A, *et al.* The ADP-ribose-1″-monophosphatase domains of severe acute respiratory syndrome coronavirus and human coronavirus 229E mediate resistance to antiviral interferon responses. J Gen Virol 2011; 92(8): 1899-905. [http://dx.doi.org/10.1099/vir.0.031856-0] [PMID: 21525212]

[42] Burgess HM, Depledge DP, Thompson L, *et al.* Targeting the m ^{6} A RNA modification pathway blocks SARS-CoV-2 and HCoV-OC43 replication. Genes Dev 2021; 35(13-14): 1005-19. [http://dx.doi.org/10.1101/gad.348320.121] [PMID: 34168039]

[43] Jaimes JA, André NM, Chappie JS, Millet JK, Whittaker GR. Phylogenetic analysis and structural modeling of SARS-CoV-2 spike protein reveals an evolutionary distinct and proteolytically sensitive activation loop. J Mol Biol 2020; 432(10): 3309-25. [http://dx.doi.org/10.1016/j.jmb.2020.04.009] [PMID: 32320687]

[44] Song G, He W, Callaghan S, *et al.* Cross-reactive serum and memory B-cell responses to spike protein in SARS-CoV-2 and endemic coronavirus infection. Nat Commun 2021; 12(1): 2938. [http://dx.doi.org/10.1038/s41467-021-23074-3] [PMID: 34011939]

[45] Siu KL, Chan CP, Kok KH, C-Y Woo P, Jin D-Y. Comparative analysis of the activation of unfolded protein response by spike proteins of severe acute respiratory syndrome coronavirus and human coronavirus HKU1. Cell Biosci 2014; 4(1): 3. [http://dx.doi.org/10.1186/2045-3701-4-3] [PMID: 24383941]

[46] Zhang N, Jiang S, Du L. Current advancements and potential strategies in the development of MERS-CoV vaccines. Expert Rev Vaccines 2014; 13(6): 761-74. [http://dx.doi.org/10.1586/14760584.2014.912134] [PMID: 24766432]

[47] Jangra M, Saxena A. Significance of physiotherapy in "SARS-CoV-2/COVID-19: An Epidemic". Ann Thorac Med 2020; 15(3): 179-80. [http://dx.doi.org/10.4103/atm.ATM_169_20] [PMID: 32831942]

[48] Zhu X, Liu S, Wang X, *et al.* Contribution of porcine aminopeptidase N to porcine deltacoronavirus infection. Emerg Microbes Infect 2018; 7(1): 1-13. [http://dx.doi.org/10.1038/s41426-018-0068-3] [PMID: 29636467]

[49] Mitrasinovic PM. Prediction of single point mutations in human coronavirus and their effects on binding to 9-O-acetylated sialic acid and hidroxychloroquine. Acta Chim Slov 2020; 67(3): 949-56. [http://dx.doi.org/10.17344/acsi.2020.6009] [PMID: 33533428]

[50] Verdecchia P, Cavallini C, Spanevello A, Angeli F. The pivotal link between ACE2 deficiency and SARS-CoV-2 infection. Eur J Intern Med 2020; 76: 14-20. [http://dx.doi.org/10.1016/j.ejim.2020.04.037] [PMID: 32336612]

[51] Huang IC, Bosch BJ, Li F, *et al.* SARS coronavirus, but not human coronavirus NL63, utilizes cathepsin L to infect ACE2-expressing cells. J Biol Chem 2006; 281(6): 3198-203. [http://dx.doi.org/10.1074/jbc.M508381200] [PMID: 16339146]

[52] Schwegmann-Weßels C, Herrler G. Sialic acids as receptor determinants for coronaviruses. Glycoconj

J 2006; 23(1-2): 51-8.
[http://dx.doi.org/10.1007/s10719-006-5437-9] [PMID: 16575522]

[53] Wang N, Shi X, Jiang L, *et al.* Structure of MERS-CoV spike receptor-binding domain complexed with human receptor DPP4. Cell Res 2013; 23(8): 986-93.
[http://dx.doi.org/10.1038/cr.2013.92] [PMID: 23835475]

[54] Corman VM, Baldwin HJ, Tateno AF, *et al.* Evidence for an ancestral association of human coronavirus 229E with bats. J Virol 2015; 89(23): 11858-70.
[http://dx.doi.org/10.1128/JVI.01755-15] [PMID: 26378164]

[55] Jacomy H, Fragoso G, Almazan G, Mushynski WE, Talbot PJ. Human coronavirus OC43 infection induces chronic encephalitis leading to disabilities in BALB/C mice. Virology 2006; 349(2): 335-46.
[http://dx.doi.org/10.1016/j.virol.2006.01.049] [PMID: 16527322]

[56] Liu SL, Saif LJ, Weiss SR, Su L. No credible evidence supporting claims of the laboratory engineering of SARS-CoV-2. Emerg Microbes Infect 2020; 9(1): 505-7.
[http://dx.doi.org/10.1080/22221751.2020.1733440] [PMID: 32102621]

[57] Woo PCY, Lau SKP, Li KSM, *et al.* Molecular diversity of coronaviruses in bats. Virology 2006; 351(1): 180-7.
[http://dx.doi.org/10.1016/j.virol.2006.02.041] [PMID: 16647731]

[58] Stout AE, Millet JK, Stanhope MJ, Whittaker GR. Furin cleavage sites in the spike proteins of bat and rodent coronaviruses: Implications for virus evolution and zoonotic transfer from rodent species. One Health 2021; 13: 100282.
[http://dx.doi.org/10.1016/j.onehlt.2021.100282] [PMID: 34179330]

[59] Yang L, Wu Z, Ren X, *et al.* MERS-related betacoronavirus in Vespertilio superans bats, China. Emerg Infect Dis 2014; 20(7): 1260-2.
[http://dx.doi.org/10.3201/eid2007.140318] [PMID: 24960574]

[60] Wahl A, Gralinski LE, Johnson CE, *et al.* SARS-CoV-2 infection is effectively treated and prevented by EIDD-2801. Nature 2021; 591(7850): 451-7.
[http://dx.doi.org/10.1038/s41586-021-03312-w] [PMID: 33561864]

[61] Stadler K, Masignani V, Eickmann M, *et al.* SARS — beginning to understand a new virus. Nat Rev Microbiol 2003; 1(3): 209-18.
[http://dx.doi.org/10.1038/nrmicro775] [PMID: 15035025]

[62] Rastogi M, Pandey N, Shukla A, Singh SK. SARS coronavirus 2: from genome to infectome. Respir Res 2020; 21(1): 318.
[http://dx.doi.org/10.1186/s12931-020-01581-z] [PMID: 33261606]

[63] Vennema H, Godeke GJ, Rossen JW, *et al.* Nucleocapsid-independent assembly of coronavirus-like particles by co-expression of viral envelope protein genes. EMBO J 1996; 15(8): 2020-8.
[http://dx.doi.org/10.1002/j.1460-2075.1996.tb00553.x] [PMID: 8617249]

[64] Malik YA. Properties of coronavirus and SARS-CoV-2. Malays J Pathol 2020; 42(1): 3-11.
[PMID: 32342926]

[65] Narayanan K, Chen CJ, Maeda J, Makino S. Nucleocapsid-independent specific viral RNA packaging *via* viral envelope protein and viral RNA signal. J Virol 2003; 77(5): 2922-7.
[http://dx.doi.org/10.1128/JVI.77.5.2922-2927.2003] [PMID: 12584316]

[66] Ganesh B, Rajakumar T, Malathi M, *et al.* Epidemiology and pathobiology of SARS-CoV-2 (COVID-19) in comparison with SARS, MERS: An updated overview of current knowledge and future perspectives. Clin Epidemiol Glob Health 2021; 10: 100694.
[http://dx.doi.org/10.1016/j.cegh.2020.100694] [PMID: 33462564]

[67] Singh N, Decroly E, Khatib AM, Villoutreix BO. Structure-based drug repositioning over the human TMPRSS2 protease domain: search for chemical probes able to repress SARS-CoV-2 Spike protein cleavages. Eur J Pharm Sci 2020; 153: 105495.

[http://dx.doi.org/10.1016/j.ejps.2020.105495] [PMID: 32730844]

[68] Davidson AM, Wysocki J, Batlle D. Interaction of sars-cov-2 and other coronavirus with ace (angiotensin-converting enzyme)-2 as their main receptor: therapeutic implications. Hypertension 2020; 76(5): 1339-49. [http://dx.doi.org/10.1161/HYPERTENSIONAHA.120.15256] [PMID: 32851855]

[69] Noor R. Antiviral drugs against severe acute respiratory syndrome coronavirus 2 infection triggering the coronavirus disease-19 pandemic. Tzu-Chi Med J 2021; 33(1): 7-12. [http://dx.doi.org/10.4103/tcmj.tcmj_100_20] [PMID: 33505872]

[70] Maier HJ, Bickerton E, Britton P. Coronaviruses: methods and protocols. Coronaviruses Methods Protoc 2015; 1282(1): 1-282.

[71] Reguera J, Mudgal G, Santiago C, Casasnovas JM. A structural view of coronavirus–receptor interactions. Virus Res 2014; 194: 3-15. [http://dx.doi.org/10.1016/j.virusres.2014.10.005] [PMID: 25451063]

[72] Das PB. The glycoproteins of porcine reproductive and respiratory syndrome virus and their role in. Infect Immun 2010.

[73] Imbert I, Snijder EJ, Dimitrova M, Guillemot JC, Lécine P, Canard B. The SARS-Coronavirus PLnc domain of nsp3 as a replication/transcription scaffolding protein. Virus Res 2008; 133(2): 136-48. [http://dx.doi.org/10.1016/j.virusres.2007.11.017] [PMID: 18255185]

[74] Romano M, Ruggiero A, Squeglia F, Maga G, Berisio R. A structural view of sars-cov-2 rna replication machinery: rna synthesis, proofreading and final capping. Cells 2020; 9(5): 1267. [http://dx.doi.org/10.3390/cells9051267] [PMID: 32443810]

[75] Perrier A, Bonnin A, Desmarets L, *et al.* The C-terminal domain of the MERS coronavirus M protein contains a *trans*-Golgi network localization signal. J Biol Chem 2019; 294(39): 14406-21. [http://dx.doi.org/10.1074/jbc.RA119.008964] [PMID: 31399512]

[76] Ng ML, Tan SH, See EE, Ooi EE, Ling AE. Proliferative growth of SARS coronavirus in Vero E6 cells. J Gen Virol 2003; 84(12): 3291-303. [http://dx.doi.org/10.1099/vir.0.19505-0] [PMID: 14645910]

[77] Christian MD, Loutfy M, McDonald LC, *et al.* Possible SARS coronavirus transmission during cardiopulmonary resuscitation. Emerg Infect Dis 2004; 10(2): 287-93. [http://dx.doi.org/10.3201/eid1002.030700] [PMID: 15030699]

[78] Zhang W, Zhao Y, Zhang F, *et al.* The use of anti-inflammatory drugs in the treatment of people with severe coronavirus disease 2019 (COVID-19): The Perspectives of clinical immunologists from China. Clin Immunol 2020; 214: 108393. [http://dx.doi.org/10.1016/j.clim.2020.108393] [PMID: 32222466]

[79] Dhama K, Sharun K, Tiwari R, *et al.* COVID-19, an emerging coronavirus infection: advances and prospects in designing and developing vaccines, immunotherapeutics, and therapeutics. Hum Vaccin Immunother 2020; 16(6): 1232-8. [http://dx.doi.org/10.1080/21645515.2020.1735227] [PMID: 32186952]

[80] Wang D, Li Z, Liu Y. An overview of the safety, clinical application and antiviral research of the COVID-19 therapeutics. J Infect Public Health 2020; 13(10): 1405-14. [http://dx.doi.org/10.1016/j.jiph.2020.07.004] [PMID: 32684351]

[81] Furuta Y, Gowen BB, Takahashi K, Shiraki K, Smee DF, Barnard DL. Favipiravir (T-705), a novel viral RNA polymerase inhibitor. Antiviral Res 2013; 100(2): 446-54. [http://dx.doi.org/10.1016/j.antiviral.2013.09.015] [PMID: 24084488]

[82] Shah B, Modi P, Sagar SR. *In silico* studies on therapeutic agents for COVID-19: Drug repurposing approach. Life Sci 2020; 252: 117652. [http://dx.doi.org/10.1016/j.lfs.2020.117652] [PMID: 32278693]

[83] Ou T, Mou H, Zhang L, Ojha A, Choe H, Farzan M. Hydroxychloroquine-mediated inhibition of SARS-CoV-2 entry is attenuated by TMPRSS2. PLoS Pathog 2021; 17(1): e1009212. [http://dx.doi.org/10.1371/journal.ppat.1009212] [PMID: 33465165]

[84] Kelleni M. NSAIDs/nitazoxanide/azithromycin immunomodulatory protocol used in adults, geriatric, pediatric, pregnant, and immunocompromised COVID-19 patients: a prospective observational study and case-series. Can J Med 2021; 3(3): 121-43.

[85] Saha A, Sharma AR, Bhattacharya M, Sharma G, Lee SS, Chakraborty C. Probable molecular mechanism of remdesivir for the treatment of COVID-19: need to know more. Arch Med Res 2020; 51(6): 585-6. [http://dx.doi.org/10.1016/j.arcmed.2020.05.001] [PMID: 32439198]

[86] Li J, Zhang C, Wu Z, Wang G, Zhao H. The Mechanism and Clinical Outcome of patients with Corona Virus Disease 2019 Whose Nucleic Acid Test has changed from negative to positive, and the therapeutic efficacy of Favipiravir: A structured summary of a study protocol for a randomised controlled trial. Trials 2020; 21(1): 488. [http://dx.doi.org/10.1186/s13063-020-04430-y] [PMID: 32503657]

[87] Ye XT, Luo YL, Xia SC, *et al.* Clinical efficacy of lopinavir/ritonavir in the treatment of Coronavirus disease 2019. Eur Rev Med Pharmacol Sci 2020; 24(6): 3390-6. [PMID: 32271456]

[88] Satarker S, Ahuja T, Banerjee M, *et al.* Hydroxychloroquine in COVID-19: potential mechanism of action against SARS-CoV-2. Curr Pharmacol Rep 2020; 6(5): 203-11. [http://dx.doi.org/10.1007/s40495-020-00231-8] [PMID: 32864299]

[89] Khatri M, Mago P. Nitazoxanide/Camostat combination for COVID-19: An unexplored potential therapy. Chemical Biology Letters 2020; 7(3): 192-6.

[90] Rizzo E. Ivermectin, antiviral properties and COVID-19: a possible new mechanism of action. Naunyn Schmiedebergs Arch Pharmacol 2020; 393(7): 1153-6. [http://dx.doi.org/10.1007/s00210-020-01902-5] [PMID: 32462282]

[91] Firandi A, Hasmono D. Effectiveness of Antiviral Drugs as Covid-19 Therapy. Journal of Tropical Pharmacy and Chemistry 2021; 5(3): 270-9. [http://dx.doi.org/10.25026/jtpc.v5i3.291]

[92] Öztürk Ö, Bağlan V, Kaya O, *et al.* Effectiveness of Favıpıravır prior to Admission to the Intensive Care Unit in COVID-19 Pneumonia. Respiratory Case Reports. 2020; 9(3).

[93] Singh AK, Singh A, Shaikh A, Singh R, Misra A. Chloroquine and hydroxychloroquine in the treatment of COVID-19 with or without diabetes: A systematic search and a narrative review with a special reference to India and other developing countries. Diabetes Metab Syndr 2020; 14(3): 241-6. [http://dx.doi.org/10.1016/j.dsx.2020.03.011] [PMID: 32247211]

[94] Cavalli G, De Luca G, Campochiaro C, *et al.* Interleukin-1 blockade with high-dose anakinra in patients with COVID-19, acute respiratory distress syndrome, and hyperinflammation: a retrospective cohort study. Lancet Rheumatol 2020; 2(6): e325-31. [http://dx.doi.org/10.1016/S2665-9913(20)30127-2] [PMID: 32501454]

[95] Hache G, Rolain JM, Gautret P, Deharo C, Brouqui P, Raoult D. Combination of hydroxychloroquine plus azithromycin as potential treatment for COVID 19 patients: pharmacology, safety profile, drug interactions and management of toxicity. 2020; 22.

[96] Mani JS, Johnson JB, Steel JC, *et al.* Natural product-derived phytochemicals as potential agents against coronaviruses: A review. Virus Res 2020; 284: 197989. [http://dx.doi.org/10.1016/j.virusres.2020.197989] [PMID: 32360300]

[97] Zhao L, Zhao Y, Wei J, Liu Z, Li C, Kang W. Antibacterial Mechanism of Dihydrotanshinone I. Nat Prod Commun 2021; 16(2): 1934578X2199615. [http://dx.doi.org/10.1177/1934578X21996158]

[98] Cai Y, Xu W, Gu C, *et al.* Griffithsin with a broad-spectrum antiviral activity by binding glycans in viral glycoprotein exhibits strong synergistic effect in combination with a pan-coronavirus fusion inhibitor targeting SARS-CoV-2 spike S2 subunit. Virol Sin 2020; 35(6): 857-60. [http://dx.doi.org/10.1007/s12250-020-00305-3] [PMID: 33052520]

[99] Du HX, Zhu JQ, Chen J, Zhou HF, Yang JH, Wan HT. Revealing the therapeutic targets and molecular mechanisms of emodin-treated coronavirus disease 2019 *via* a systematic study of network pharmacology. Aging (Albany NY) 2021; 13(11): 14571-89. [http://dx.doi.org/10.18632/aging.203098] [PMID: 34088885]

[100] Wang SC, Chen Y, Wang YC, *et al.* Tannic acid suppresses SARS-CoV-2 as a dual inhibitor of the viral main protease and the cellular TMPRSS2 protease. Am J Cancer Res 2020; 10(12): 4538-46. [PMID: 33415017]

[101] Umar HI, Siraj B, Ajayi A, Jimoh TO, Chukwuemeka PO. Molecular docking studies of some selected gallic acid derivatives against five non-structural proteins of novel coronavirus. J Genet Eng Biotechnol 2021; 19(1): 16. [http://dx.doi.org/10.1186/s43141-021-00120-7] [PMID: 33492492]

[102] Balkrishna A. POKHREL S, Singh J, Varshney A. Withanone from Withania somnifera may inhibit novel coronavirus (COVID-19) entry by disrupting interactions between viral S-protein receptor binding domain and host ACE2 receptor. 2020.

[103] Kim JY, Kim YI, Park SJ, Kim IK, Choi YK, Kim SH. Safe, high-throughput screening of natural compounds of MERS-CoV entry inhibitors using a pseudovirus expressing MERS-CoV spike protein. Int J Antimicrob Agents 2018; 52(5): 730-2. [http://dx.doi.org/10.1016/j.ijantimicag.2018.05.003] [PMID: 29772395]

[104] Barre A, Van Damme EJM, Simplicien M, *et al.* Man-specific lectins from plants, fungi, algae and cyanobacteria, as potential blockers for SARS-CoV, MERS-CoV and SARS-CoV-2 (COVID-19) coronaviruses: Biomedical perspectives. Cells 2021; 10(7): 1619. [http://dx.doi.org/10.3390/cells10071619] [PMID: 34203435]

[105] Coelho C, Gallo G, Campos CB, Hardy L, Würtele M. Biochemical screening for SARS-CoV-2 main protease inhibitors. PLoS One 2020; 15(10): e0240079. [http://dx.doi.org/10.1371/journal.pone.0240079] [PMID: 33022015]

[106] Ma Q, Wang Z, Chen R, *et al.* Effect of Jinzhen granule on two coronaviruses: The novel SARS-Co--2 and the HCoV-229E and the evidences for their mechanisms of action. Phytomedicine 2022; 95: 153874. [http://dx.doi.org/10.1016/j.phymed.2021.153874] [PMID: 34923232]

[107] Kumar V, Dhanjal JK, Kaul SC, Wadhwa R, Sundar D. Withanone and caffeic acid phenethyl ester are predicted to interact with main protease (M^{pro}) of SARS-CoV-2 and inhibit its activity. J Biomol Struct Dyn 2021; 39(11): 3842-54. [http://dx.doi.org/10.1080/07391102.2020.1772108] [PMID: 32431217]

[108] Singh VK, Mishra A, Singh S, *et al.* Emerging prevention and treatment strategies to control COVID-19. Pathogens 2020; 9(6): 501. [http://dx.doi.org/10.3390/pathogens9060501] [PMID: 32585805]

CHAPTER 2

COVID-19: Sign, Symptoms and Transmission

Saket Singh Chandel[1,*], **Deepshikha Verma**[2] and **Vipinchandra Bhaskarrao Pande**[3]

[1] *Department of Pharmacology, Dr. C. V. Raman Institute of Pharmacy, Dr. C. V. Raman University, Bilaspur-495113, Chhattisgarh, India*

[2] *Institute of Pharmaceutical Sciences, Guru Ghasidas Vishwavidyalaya, Koni, Bilaspur-495009, Chhattisgarh, India*

[3] *Department of Pharmacy, Mandsaur University, Mandsaur-458001, Madhya Pradesh, India*

Abstract: COVID-19, which is caused by SARS-CoV-2, was first reported in Wuhan, China in late 2019. Till date, over 12.1 million people have contracted the disease across 221 countries in the world. The global fatality rate is about 6.2% thus far, and as of May 26th 2020, the highest confirmed cases were recorded in the USA, Brazil, Russia, Spain, UK, Italy and France. Several attempts to fight against the virus are taken by the World Health Organization (WHO) as well as other health agencies in various countries with reported confirmed cases. The present study has reviewed COVID-19 with respect to the clinical symptoms and signs, as well as factors that could exacerbate COVID-19 condition and transmission amongst people. Recent reports and studies have found the disease status to be of the predominantly mild condition and to a lesser extent, a critical/severe status. COVID-19 presents several clinical manifestations with symptoms such as fever, dry cough, fatigue, dizziness, anorexia, headache, expectoration, dyspnea, chest tightness, abdominal pain, diarrhea and nausea. Studies have observed age, obesity, smoking and drinking habit, immune system condition, human selectivity and reactivity as factors that can aggravate the disease condition, while poverty, fake news, non-validated scientific claims, and perception/illiteracy have been reported as risk components that could enhance the transmission of the viral infection. This study concludes by suggesting the appropriate methods to combat the factors discussed.

Keywords: Co-Morbidities, COVID-19, Global Pandemic, Immune System, Public Health, SARS-CoV-2.

* **Corresponding author Saket Singh Chandel:** Department of Pharmacology, Dr. C. V. Raman Institute of Pharmacy, Dr. C. V. Raman University, Bilaspur-495113, Chhattisgarh, India, Mobile: +919827181552; Email Id: singhpharma@gmail.com

1. INTRODUCTION

In early January 2020, there were several global news concerning the emergence of a novel coronavirus in Wuhan, Hubei Province, China. Prior to that time, specifically towards mid-December 2019, there were cases of unknown pneumonia in the province reported. It rapidly became a major source of concern to the Chinese Government and its health institutions. Consequently, an etiological study was launched to curtail its spread. According to Kakodkar *et al.* (2020), China's CDC discovered a virus called novel coronavirus 2019 (2019-nCoV) and it was colloquially referred to as "Wuhan Coronavirus" on 7th January, 2020 [1].

The causative agent responsible for the disease was identified as Severe Acute Respiratory Syndrome (SARS-CoV-2) by scientists. By the end of January 2020, WHO had declared 2019-nCoV a public health emergency. The cases were increasing in China, before the virus had spread to other nations and territories across various continents of the world. During this period, the WHO had closely monitored the situation and the name of the disease was given as Coronavirus Disease 2019 with a short name of COVID-19 by 11th February, 2020. Authors had attributed the renaming of the "Wuhan Coronavirus" as SARS-CoV-2 as an attempt to de-stigmatize the association of the virus with respect to the geographic locality and in relation to the disease symptomatology [1]. By 11th March 2020, COVID-19 was declared a global pandemic.

Presently, the disease has spread to over 221 countries and territories. The major means of the virus transmission include person to person, making contact with SARS-Cov-2 contaminated surfaces as well as having exposure to and inhalation of droplets released by SARS-Cov-2 patients through aerosolization. The disease has been reported to affect the respiratory tracts which would lead to coughing, sneezing, difficulty in breathing or shortness of breath and pneumonia among others [2].

Information obtained from the Worldometer website as of March 16, 2021, 10:38 GMT has shown that over 12.1 million people have contracted the disease across 221 countries in the world to date. The total numbers of confirmed deaths, recovered and discharged cases were 2,672,766; 100,107,434 and 97,434,668 respectively. Among the active cases currently (20,687,790), 99.6% and 0.4% are in mild and critical conditions, respectively. Presently (Till 16th March, 2021), the number of nations with the highest cases are in this order USA (30,138,586), Brazil (11,525,477), India (11,409,831), Russia (4,400,045), UK (4,263, 527), France (4,078,133), Italy (3,238,394) and Spain (3,195,062), while the countries with the highest death rates are in the order; USA (548,013), Brazil (279,602),

Mexico (194,944), India (158,892), UK (125,580), Italy (102,499), Russia (92,494), France (90,762), Germany (74,115) and Spain (72,424). China is ranked as the 86th nation with the highest number of confirmed cases (90,062) while India and Nigeria are ranked 3rd and 73rd, respectively. India had 11,146,371 confirmed cases, 158,892 deaths, 11,027,543 discharged cases, 223,396 active cases and 8,944 cases in critical condition, while the most populated nation in Africa (Nigeria) had 160,895 confirmed cases, 2,016 deaths, 145,752 discharged cases, 13,127 active cases and 10 in critical condition [2].

A large number of deaths have been recorded as a result of the global pandemic of COVID-19 in which most of the deaths were individuals with underlying health conditions. It is opined that chronic medical conditions would commonly occur in combination which is also known as comorbidities [3]. Researchers have reported that comorbidity is related to adverse health effects, more intricate clinical management and increased cost of health care. It is difficult to accurately define the relationship between a disease and its comorbidities [4]. Furthermore, the nature and prevalence of the comorbidities are mainly swayed by their epidemiology in the patients' area of origin. Most comorbidities of a disease often influence its clinical manifestations and may cause uncertainties in their diagnosis.

Effective management of chronic medical conditions with comorbidities is accrued with multifaceted treatment procedures, therefore, entails suitable self-care by the patients of all comorbid conditions. This can be made possible by understanding the underlying mechanisms, the causative agent of the diseases as well as their interactions [4]. The coexistence of other infectious comorbidities in patients with life-threatening ailments has been recorded in the literature. Studies have shown that most people that had died from COVID-19 had suffered from other health conditions. The comorbidity rate of COVID-19 patients is at least 74.4% and 58.8% of it are from various parts of the pandemic area [5, 6]. Some of the common health conditions associated with COVID-19 include chronic obstructive pulmonary/lung disease, cardiovascular diseases, diabetes, hypertension, chronic liver and kidney disease, malignant tumor, and bacteria co-infection among others [7 - 12].

Therefore, this study is aimed at reviewing the factors that could aggravate the condition and transmission as well as increasing the awareness of the severity status of the disease.

2. SIGNS, SYMPTOMS AND SEVERITY STATUS OF COVID-19 PATIENTS

The clinical presentation of COVID-19 is classified into several categories. One of the categories is called "severe case" (a condition where a patient is characterized by respiratory distress syndrome with respiratory rates of ≥30BPM (Breaths Per Minute), post 5 minutes of rest, the oxygen saturation measured on finger is ≤93%, the arterial oxygen partial pressure PaO_2 is ≤300 mmHg/the inspired oxygen fraction FiO2, with dyspnea, tachypnea: ≥70BPM (<1year), ≥50BPM (≥1 year), hypoxia (oxygen saturation <92%), or >50% pulmonary involvement on imaging within 24 to 48 hours, disturbance of consciousness and feeding difficulty with signs of dehydration. Meanwhile, a critical case is a condition where a patient is characterized by respiratory failure that requires intubation [13, 14]. Another classification of COVID-19 is "mild case", which is characterized by no/mild pneumonia [15]. The final category is grouped as "moderate case". It has been reported that mild and severe cases had occurred approximately amongst 81% and 14% proportion of COVID-19 patients, respectively [16]. The information available from the Worldometer website as of 16th March, 2021, 10:38 GMT has shown that 98% and 2% of active cases are in mild and critical conditions, respectively. Most patients with mild and moderate cases often would recover, especially when they do not have existing health-threatening comorbidities [2].

Studies have shown that there are variations in the disease severity of COVID-19 patients depending on the comorbidity. For instance, it has been reported that the comorbidities of COVID-19 are in the order; cardiovascular > endocrine system > respiratory > gastrointestinal >urinary system >malignant tumor > inflammatory diseases. The authors have further reported that the disease severity is in the order; critical > severe > mild to moderate (for respiratory, cardiovascular, gastrointestinal, endocrine system, inflammatory, urinary system diseases), severe > critical > mild to moderate (for malignant tumor). It is also reported that the severity of cases observed among COVID-19 patients had respiratory infections (chronic obstructive pulmonary disease), cardiovascular diseases (hypertension, coronary heart disease) and cancer (malignant tumor). This further emphasizes that patients with comorbidities tend to develop critical or severe cases [13 - 16].

Researchers have reported signs and symptoms of COVID-19 patients based on conditions such as respiratory, digestive, systemic and neurological symptoms, with the disease severity (*viz*: mild to moderate, severe and critical condition). The authors have reported the statistical deviation in the severity of disease *viz*: mild to moderate, severe and critical with respect to dyspnea and chest tightness, and no significant variation with respect to dry cough, expectoration (respiratory symptoms), no significant deviation with respect to abdominal pains, nausea, vomiting and bloating, and significant difference with regard to diarrhoea (digestive symptoms), significant variations with regard to fatigue, dizziness and muscle ache, and no statistical deviation with respect to fever and headache (systemic symptoms), and unconsciousness (neurological symptoms). In short, it is believed that fever, dry cough and fatigue are the predominant symptoms; while fever, dizziness, muscle ache, expectoration, dyspnea, and chest tightness on admission are also found to influence patients' recovery progress in the hospital. Of all the symptoms recorded, dyspnea and unconsciousness are said to be related to mortality [17 - 20].

During the diagnosis of the disease in the laboratory, there are several abnormalities observed such as; increased enzymes level (liver, muscles, lactate, creatine kinase isoenzyme, myoglobin), decreased immunity (lymphopenia), increased levels of prolactin, ESR (erythrocyte sedimentation rate) and C-reactive protein [21]. During this process, some blood-related parameters are altered in which there is an increase in total white blood cells, neutrophils and a decrease in lymphocytes and hemoglobin (routine blood parameters), an increase in aspartate aminotransferase and alanine aminotransferase (liver function), bilateral pneumonia (computed tomography), an increase in lactate dehydrogenase, a decrease in albumin level, and an increase in the C-reactive protein and kidney function damage [21]. The authors further reported a significant variation in the status of the disease severity (mild to moderate, critical and severe). There are several aberrations which are common to COVID-19 patients during laboratory diagnosis which include hypoalbuminemia, lymphopenia, the decline in lymphocytes and neutrophils, and CD8 count, coupled with an increase in the C-reactive protein and lactate dehydrogenase. The authors also have stated that the viral load of SARS-CoV-2 from the patients' respiratory tracts is positively linked to lung disease severity. Furthermore, it is also suggested that COVID-19 is characterized by pneumonia with an aberration in chest computed tomography [21].

Different patients have shown varying symptoms of COVID-19 as age plays a significant role in determining the symptoms experienced. The common symptoms of COVID-19 reported are mentioned in Table **1** [8 - 10, 14].

Studies have reported that there are no significant variations between the mild and severe status to signs and symptoms with respect to fever, runny nose, sore throat, sputum, dyspnea, fatigue, anorexia, muscle ache, nausea, diarrhea and headache despite showing statistical deviation with respect to dry cough and chest tightness [19]. Furthermore, COVID-19 patients that had undergone surgery also had shown signs and symptoms such as fever, fatigue, dry cough, dyspnea, myalgia or arthralgia, expectoration, dizziness or headache, pharyngula, anorexia, nausea, diarrhea and abdominal pain during the surgical process. There have been more signs and symptoms reported among patients in intensive care units when compared to their counterparts in non-intensive care units [21].

Table 1. Clinical manifestations and physical signs and Symptoms of COVID-19.

Signs and Symptoms	Lang Wang [10],	Lei S [19],	Meng Y [11],	Xu XW [12],	Zhang J [13],	Guan W [14],	Huang C [15],	Liu Y [8],	Wang D [9],	Zheng J [21],
Age	49.16 years (mean)	55 years (median); 43-63 years (Inter quartile range)	56.7 years (mean)	41 years (median); 32-52 years (Inter quartile range)	16-95 years (Range); 55.6 years (Median)	47.0 years (median); 35.0–58.0 years (Inter quartile range)	49·0 years (median); 41–58 years (Inter quartile range)	20-83 years (Range); 57 years (Median); 55 years (Mean)	56 years (Median); 42-68 years (Inter quartile range)	57 years (Median); 25-87 years (range)
Gender: Male Female	49 51	41.2 58.8	51.19 48.81	58 44	48.4% 51.6%	58.1 41.9	73 27	44.53 55.57	54.3 45.7	50.7 49.3
Date	Jan 1 to Feb 6, 2020	Jan 1 to Feb 5,2020	Jan 16 and Feb 4, 2020	Jan 10 to Jan 26, 2020	January 11 to Feb 6, 2020	Dec 11, 2019 and Jan 31, 2020	Dec 16, 2019, to Jan 2, 2020	Dec 30, 2019 to Jan 24, 2020	Jan 1 to Feb2, 2020	Jan 16 to Feb 3, 2020
Study region	Renmin Hospital of Wuhan University	Renmin Hospital, Zhong nan Hospital, Tongji Hospital and Central Hospital in Wuhan	Tongji Hospital in Wuhan, China	Zhejiang province	Renmin Hospital of Wuhan University	National Health Commission	JinYintan Hospital (Wuhan, China)	Nine tertiary hospitals in Hubei province	Zhong nan Hospital of Wuhan University	Zhong nan hospital of Wuhan University
Cough	53	52.9	72	81	61.8	67.8	76	48.2	59.4	75
Expectoration	27.5	32.4	41.7	56	25.0	-	-	4.4	26.8	-
Dyspnea	40.8	44.1	35.1	-	24.3	-	55	19.0	31	36.7**
Chest tightness	26	-	-	-	23.2	-	-	-	2	-
Pharyngalgia	12.7	20.6	4.2	-	-	-	-	-	17.4	-
Pharyngeal hypereramia	-	-	1.8	-	-	-	-	-	-	-
Throat congestion	-	-	-	-	-	1.7	-	-	-	-
Nasal congestion	-	-	-	-	-	4.8	-	-	-	-
Sore throat	-	-	-	-	-	13.9	-	-	-	-
Sputum production	-	-		-	-	33.7	-	-	-	-
Shortness of breath	-	-	-	-	-	18.7	-	-	-	-

(Table 1) cont.....

Signs and Symptoms	Lang Wang [10],	Lei S [19],	Meng Y [11],	Xu XW [12],	Zhang J [13],	Guan W [14],	Huang C [15],	Liu Y [8],	Wang D [9],	Zheng J [21],
Thoracodynia	-	-	7.1	-	-	-	-	-	-	-
Gastrointestinal	-	-	-	-	-	-	-	-	-	39.6
Abdominal pain	-	2.9	4.2	-	0.8	-	-	-	2.2	5.8
Diarrhea	-	5.9	26.2	8	9.2	3.8	3.0	8.0	10.1	12.9
Nausea	3.8	8.8	10.7	-	4.7	5.0***	-	-	10.1	17.3
Vomiting	-	-	8.9	-	2.6	-	-	-	3.6	
Bloating/ belching	-	-	-	-	1.2	-	-	-	-	5.0
Fever	92	91.2	92.9	77	9.5	-	98.0	81.8	98.6	91.7
Fatigue	39.9	73.5	38.7	52*	31.4	38.1	44*	32.1*	69.6	75.0
Myalgia	4.7	-	28.7	-	-	14.9	-	-	34.8	-
Dizziness	3.8	-	4.2	-	3.5	-	-	-	9.4	-
Headache	3.5	23.5****	13.1	34	3.0	13.6	8.0	9.5	6.5	-
Muscle ache	-	-	-	-	9.3	-	-	-	-	-
Unconsciousness	-	-	-	-	1.5	-	-	-	-	-
Hemoptysis	-	-	1.8	3		0.9	5.0	5.1	-	-
Heart palpation	-	-	-	-	-	-	-	7.3	-	-
Anorexia	27.8	14.7	8.9	-	-	-	-	-	39.9	12.2
Emesis	-	-	-	-	-	-	-	-	-	5.0
Tonsil swelling	-	-	-	-	-	2.1	-	-	-	-
Enlargement of the lymph nodes	-	-	-	-	-	0.2	-	-	-	-
Conjunctival congestion	-	-	-	-	-	0.8	-	-	-	-
Rashes	-	-	-	-	-	0.2	-	-	-	-
Chills	-	-	-	-	-	11.5	-	-	-	-

*Treated as myalgia or fatigue; ** treated as dyspnea or chest tightness; *** treated as vomiting or nausea; **** treated as dizziness or headache.

Majority of COVID-19 patients would often experience mild to moderate symptoms and they are able to recover fully without any form of a particular treatment. The most common symptoms among patients in critical conditions are often based on their underlying medical conditions. Based on the severity of COVID-19 cases, 27.4% were given oxygen therapy, 34.5% had used nasal or face mask oxygen, 42.9% had received high-flow nasal oxygen therapy, 20.2% were kept in noninvasive ventilation and 1.2% had to be intubated with invasive mechanical ventilation. There are also patients that have been treated with extracorporeal membrane oxygenation. The authors also have highlighted that age is not a factor that would influence intubation [5].

The signs and symptoms of the disease would begin to manifest within 1-14 days, depending on the patient's immune system. During this extensive period, there have been circumstances whereby patients have not shown any signs or symptoms (asymptomatic). The median time of exposure to the onset of illness of SARS-Cov-2 in Zhejiang province was 4 days (interquartile range 3-5 days) and from the onset of symptoms to the first hospital admission, it was 2 days (1-4 days) [20]. Moreover, it is said that 4.99 days time was the period from illness onset to dyspnea [21].

Complications resulting from COVID-19 are stated in Table **2**. The most common complications include acute respiratory distress syndrome, acute cardiac injury, acute kidney injury, arrhythmia and shock. Therefore, performing surgery on COVID-19 carriers may result in complications. Acute respiratory disease syndrome, shock, secondary infection, arrhythmia, acute cardiac injury and acute kidney injury are higher among patients in the intensive care unit compared to their counterparts in the non-intensive care units [5].

Table 2. Common complications resulting from COVID-19 (Values expressed as a percentage).

Common Complications	Guan W, [14]	Lei S, [19]	Lang Wang, [10]	Huang C, [15]	Tan SC, [20]
Acute respiratory distress syndrome	3.4	32.40	21.00	29	28.36
Acute respiratory injury	-	-	-	-	2.34
RNAaemia	-	-	-	15	1.75
Cycle threshold of RNAaemia	-	-	-	34·7–35·1	-
Disseminated intravascular coagulation	0.1	-	-	-	-
Rhabdomyolysis	0.1	-	-	-	-
Acute cardiac injury*		14.70	21.00	12	7.89
Acute kidney injury	0.5	5.90	8.1	7	7.60
Secondary infection	-	29.40	-	10	1.17
Shock	1.1	29.40	5.9	7	5.85
Arrhythmia		23.50	10.40		6.73
Shock Hyperglycemia	-	-	-	-	5.26
Hepatic insufficiency/liver dysfunction	-	-	-	-	4.97
Liver Enzyme Abnormalities	-	-	28.7	-	-
Hospital acquired/Ventilator associated pneumonia	-	-	-	-	2.34
Gastrointestinal hemorrhage	-	-	-	-	0.58
Cardiac failure or insufficiency	-	-	17.4	-	0.29
Pneumothorax	-	-	-	-	0.29

(Table 2) cont.....

Renal insufficiency	-	-	-	-	0.58
Urinary tract infection	-	-	-	-	0.29
Bacteremia	-	-	-	-	0.29
Bacterial Infection	-	-	42.8	-	

3. FACTORS THAT AGGRAVATE COVID-19 CONDITION

3.1. Age

Age group is associated with chronic illnesses due to diminishing of tiny molecules that would attack any invading viruses. Furthermore, with age and some chronic medical conditions, attacking micro RNA numbers would decrease, reducing their ability to respond to viruses. In this study, scientists assessed the RNA sequence of two coronaviruses namely; SARS-2002 and SARS –CoV-2 [24]. According to the study, SARS-848 Micro RNA targeted the genome, much in the same manner as SARS-COV-19–873 Micro RNA had targeted the genome [24].

According to the studies performed, about 558 of the micro RNAs fighting SARS are also present in SARS-COV-2, while SARS-COV2 and SARS have unique micro RNAs 393 and 290 respectively [24]. Many of these tiny RNA molecules are known to diminish with age and other underlying medical conditions such as diabetes mellitus and coronary artery disease. The decrease in the numbers of micro RNAs leads to an increase in death rates, therefore, making the individuals more prone to risks. Micro RNAs with an affinity for SARS-CoV-2 is less-protected in people with coronary artery disease, especially the elderly [26].

3.2. Obesity

The oxygen capacity of lungs depends on fat levels and it is affected by obesity (higher levels of fat in the chest and belly). Reduction in breathing capacity leads to respiratory distress in patients with COVID-19 [25].

Obesity also affects the immune system and alters various inflammatory levels similar to COVID-19 patients. Due to this, individuals with obesity have a higher possibility to contract COVID-19 infection. Furthermore, fat tissues act as vast reservoirs for macrophage and T cell after infection with COVID-19. Whilst it is already known that obese individuals are at risk of chronic ailments, the body mass index (BMI) has been identified to portend adverse health hazards in the event of contracting the novel coronavirus. Most notably, increasing BMI is also associated with critical or severe COVID-19 health cases [25].

3.3. Smoking

Smoking is believed to extend the danger of being infected with the novel coronavirus. Studies have shown marked and reasonably increased ACE2 gene expression in the lungs of the former and some current smokers when compared to non-smokers. Most importantly, the ACE2 gene was observed in specific cells that had shown the history and location of smoking [26]. Smokers have high ACE2 receptors in their lungs as well as high goblet and club cells in LRT compared to non-smokers [27]. In 1999, as reported by the "American journal of respiratory and critical care medicine", the secretory cells of lungs are boosted by smoking. The numbers of secretory cells and the production of mucus had increased which lead to the respiratory depression due to coughing and sneezing [28]. Therefore, smoking may likely be a reason for the declining health situation among COVID-19 patients who are also active smokers [29 - 31].

3.4. Drinking

Alcohol consumption can increase the risk of contracting COVID-19 and worsen the impact of the virus as alcohol compromises the body's immune system and increases the risk of adverse health outcomes [32]. Alcoholic individuals generally have weak immunity (risky to communicable and non-communicable diseases) thus making them more susceptible to COVID-19. With the enforcement of home quarantine and social distancing in many parts of the world, it is observed that alcohol consumption has increased which affects behavioral changes and leads to psychotic disorders [33].

3.5. Immune System Condition

People of various age groups have different immune systems. The cause of many health problems is said to be related to weak immune systems. The immune system is a network of cells, tissues and organs that are working together to prevent infection from bacteria, parasites or fungi. The immune system however is not the same for two individuals. WHO has issued recommendations for the modification of public health and social policies as the next step of the COVID-19 response. Several policymakers have indicated that the discovery of antibodies to the COVID-19-causing SARS-CoV-2 virus could serve as the basis for an "immunity passport" or "risk-free certificate" that would allow individuals to move or return to work on the presumption that they are protected against re-infection [34]. Nevertheless, till date, there is no recovery reported from COVID-19 with antibodies. The development of immunity through natural exposure to a pathogen is usually a multi-stage cycle that takes place over 1-2 weeks. The body would mechanically respond to a virus infection with a non-specific innate reaction during which macrophages, neutrophils and nerve fiber cells would delay the virus' development and inhibit it from inflicting symptoms. Following this non-specific response, the body produces antibodies that would specifically square measure coupled to the virus. The proteins are referred to as immunoglobulins. These antibodies in the organism would conjointly develop T cells that can sense and kill bound virus-infected cells [35]. There is a possibility that antibodies within the blood would assess this cycle. Virus infection and the replication in the airway of animal tissue cells might cause high rates of virus-related pyroptosis with associated vascular discharge, as seen in SARS-CoV patients. Pyroptosis could be an extreme inflammatory pathway that always occurs with cytopathic viruses for programmed death. The subsequent inflammatory reaction is activated. Throughout SARS-CoV-2 infection, IL-1β would be a major protein discharged throughout pyroptosis. Alveolar animal tissue cells and alveolar macrophages, together with microorganism's ribonucleic acid and DAMPs would recognize a range of pattern-recognition receptors (PRRs), and alternative discharged Pathogen-associated molecular patterns (PAMPs) [36, 37]. There is a surge of native inflammation involving the secretion of IL-6, IFNα, MCP1, and T aid IP (TH1) pro-inflammatory cytokines and chemokines, in addition to the findings of the SARS-COVs and MERS-COVs [38]. The Granulocyte colony-stimulation issue (G-CSF), IP-10, MCP1 in these patients has continued to rise and it is relatively higher for the non-survivor than for the survivor. The inflammatory phagocyte proteins are (MIP1α), tumor necrosis factor and IL-6 levels. The most unmistakably, exceptionally fiery, monocyte-based FCN1 + phagocyte populace is available inside the Broncho alveolar lavage liquid in patients with genuine, in any case, not moderate COVID-19 manifestations. Furthermore, infringe blood CD-14+CD16 + has demonstrated to be extensively higher in patients with severe disease than in patients with moderate affliction [39, 40].

3.6. Human Selectivity and Reactivity

The SARS-CoV-2 belongs to the type 2 classification of coronaviruses which is highly transmissible. The current COVID-19 strain shows 17% variability from the SARS-CoV RATG13. The analysis of 103 SARS-CoV-2 genomes indicates that the evolution of the viruses is split into two (2) types, L (~70%) and S (~30%), with the L-type being the most occurring. Moreover, SARS-CoV-2 is found to bind to human ACE2 with strong affinity. Overall, they have shown stronger bonds than SARS-CoV proteins, which is likely due to natural human selection. In fact, most isolates which were obtained from patients across China,

Thailand and USA had shown increased genetic diversity of the virus among human carriers [41, 42]. Humans who are living within the vicinity of bat caves in China have been found to possess antibodies against the bat SARS-type coronaviruses [42]. Several studies have shown the prevalence of insertion/deletion polymorphisms of ACE genes. The frequency of the D allele (responsible for hereditary characteristics) of ACE genes has shown similarities between Omanis (0.71) and the other Arab groups: Emirates (0.66), Somali (0.73) and Sudan (0.64) with the D allele from the Arab group revealing the highest distribution [42]. Generally, the clinical distribution is in the following order: Africans and Arabs (0.60 – 0.70) > Caucasians (0.46 – 0.58) > Japanese (0.33 – 0.35) > Chinese (0.29) >Yanomami Indians (0.15) > Samoans (0.09), respectively. Evidently, the D alleles of various races in the world have shown reasonable differences [41]. The D allele is related to decreasing ACE2 expression in human tissue with multiple forms of D/L alleles depicting variability to geographical locations. In addition, its log has revealed a prevalence of COVID-19 ailments being inversely correlated to the D allele frequency. In spite of the possibility of selectivity and immunity that the D allele frequencies provide, the impact of immune responses on COVID-19 is yet to be known. However, studies have indeed suggested that immunity against one virus of the sarbecovirus subgenus may likely protect a person from similar viruses [42].

4. FACTORS THAT ENHANCE THE TRANSMISSION OF COVID-19

4.1. Misdiagnosis

So far, there are similarities in symptoms of COVID-19 with other diseases such as influenza, common cold (caused by rhinovirus), para-influenza, acute febrile illness and coronary obstructive pulmonary disease (Table **3**).

Table 3. Symptoms of COVID-19 in comparison with flu and the common cold [43].

Conditions	COVID-19	FLU	COMMON COLD
Incubation Period	2-14 Days	1-4 days	1-3 days
Symptoms	Gradual	Abrupt	Gradual
Cough	Common	Common	Mild to moderate
Shortness of Breath	Common	Sometimes	Mild
Fever	Common	Common	Rare
Fatigue	Common	Common	Sometimes
Runny nose	Sometimes	Sometimes	Common

4.2. Poverty

Health and poverty are integrally intertwined factors as one goes a long way towards determining the other. Several studies have highlighted the prevalence of infection and transmission of certain diseases in impoverished regions. According to WHO, approximately, there are about 1.2 billion people around the world who live in an extreme poverty (less than one dollar per day) [44]. Poverty is characterized by the lack of food, clean water, shelter, adequate sanitation, security and social protection which put these people in a situation whereby they are more vulnerable to infections. Consequently, these affected populations are often unable to enjoy even the most basic means of prevention and care. Over 40% of the world's population lives in poorly sanitized areas and more than 1 billion people have to consume unsafe sources of drinking water. Poverty in this context refers not only to money but also to skills and assets, as most poor people are usually less educated and unable to get good jobs hence, relying on menial jobs to support their families [45, 46].

Coronavirus may disproportionately hurt those who are poor and low-income earners as they are more likely to be uninsured or underinsured for medical care. Lacking resources to prepare and be protected against COVID-19 infection would make them at a higher risk of contracting and subsequently spreading the virus. The key advice from health care professionals is to avoid crowded areas and maintain at least 6 feet distance from others within public places. However, the chance of transmission would increase especially among low-income families as they are more likely to live in small quarters with multiple people sharing common utilities. Poor populations with a lack of access to health services in normal circumstances are left vulnerable during the current crisis. Subsequently, misinformation and miscommunication would disproportionally affect individuals with limited access to information channels, as they are more likely to ignore government health warnings [47].

4.3. Perception and Illiteracy

Illiteracy and low educational status are believed to be the determinant of disease spread and mortality and they are often the most prevalent in low-income countries. Illiteracy poses a big problem as the average person is not able to comprehend the implication of this worldwide pandemic. It is alarming as the majority of these people even believe that COVID-19 is a shame, especially those who are living in the rural areas of developing countries. Poor health literacy is an underestimated global public health problem [48, 49].

4.4. Asymptomatic Patients

Generally, COVID-19 illness is classified as mild, moderate, severe and asymptomatic. Asymptomatic patients who are tested positive in cluster examinations do not have any symptoms prior to testing, therefore, would enhance the transmission of the disease as they believe that they are healthy. Due to this, they have the tendency to spread the infection to other people whose immune systems have been compromised or currently utilise corticosteroids or belong to CAD/ACS/ILD/COPD. However, a recent study has reported that there is no statistical difference between the transmissibility of asymptomatic cases compared to symptomatic cases [50, 51].

4.5. Climatic Influence

The climate has been identified as one of the major supporters of human biological differences and their adaptability toward survival. Decreasing ultraviolet (UV) radiation and atmospheric oxygen have contributed to changes in human biology. The movement of surviving human species from hot-tropical Africa, which is known for increased sunlight, to the north of Europe with significantly reduced UV radiation, as well as the diversified respiration and reproductive physiological differences has been observed among those who are living within high altitudes, thereby enabling their survival and reproductive ability, even at low atmospheric oxygen [52].

An association is believed to exist between persistent metabolic sickness and physiological variation within the past human population adapted to their typical climatic environments. Consequently, the movement of tropically-adapted humans to cold-temperate regions has previously resulted in cases whereby Afro-Americans have shown a greater prevalence of hypertension, heart and kidney failures as compared to their Euro-American counterparts. This may have been due to the discrepancies between familial tropical hot climates and other comparatively chilly weather that is salt-rich. For example, different individuals would exhibit varying fragilities to disease outbreaks. Overall, the interface between culture and biology is as important as the existence of biological varieties and disparity in health responses. Hence, metabolic illnesses such as diabetes, lipid disarray and cancers amongst others have shown varying prevalences based on ethnobiological adaptabilities that are still being investigated [53, 54].

The effect of global climatic environmental hazards on human health is known to be of significant importance to man's sustenance. As such, confirmed degradation could negatively impact the increasing human population and biodiversity. The manner in which a population reacts to disease spread is dependent on climate change and adaptability to a new climate, as well as their responses which may be dependent on locality, economic expansion, adequate food supply, overall income allocation, localized environmental hygiene, public health status and available care. This is because reports have shown that the impoverished population class, infant/young children and ageing people are the most prone to health hazards. Meanwhile, adaptation to health threats, especially posed by global climate change, can take place either spontaneously or gradually, which in turn tends to prompt certain physiological reactions from the human body. Therefore, it is pertinent to ensure that sensible measures are taken to forestall or manage the impacts of climate change as it could provide us a minimal chance to carry out a preliminary assessment of alternatives for acclimatization [55].

Currently, significant meteorological changes are beginning to occur more frequently (at weekly or monthly intervals) as opposed to previous timelines which would have spanned several decades. For example, abnormal changes in climatic conditions such as ambient temperature and rainfall during a seasonal term have often resulted in the prevalence of a number of pathogens and disease-carrying organisms, leading to epidemics that often would persist until the reversal of the causative climatic parameter (WHO, 2003) [53]. Excessive heat has been reported to cause heat exhaustion and cardiovascular illness while extreme chilly temperatures can result in hypothermia and death from the cardiovascular ailment. On the other hand, instant injuries or even death often derived from more extreme weather conditions such as storms, tropical cyclones and torrential rains. While a slow-changing climate would allow time for inhabitants to adapt, individuals who are exposed to sudden climatic changes have limited time to survive. Furthermore, climatic and environmental considerations are known to kick-start the spread of illness and epidemic set-off. Even though human adenovirus (HPIV) is very similar to COVID-19 as it is often rendered inactive through the application of soap and water during hand washing, the use of antiseptics and disinfectants, HPIVs are more susceptible to environmental factors such as pH, relative humidity, temperature, amongst others. The infectivity of this virus would slow down at pH values between 7.4 and 8.0, temperatures exceeding 37°C and low humidity. However, it is worth noting that the effects of typical high temperatures and the characteristic of low humidity on the coronavirus have not been extensively studied. Moreover, the effects of recent climate or weather changes on the viral outbreak and its spread are yet to be established as well [53]. Based on research conducted, environmental factors such as thermal conditions, relative humidity and UV radiation do not slow down the spread of COVID-19 in some areas in China [52]. However, findings from this report are yet to be supported by additional meteorological information from across the globe. There is also a debate as to whether the virus would spread faster in more temperate regions. A recent study has reported that SARS-CoV-2 did not spread as efficiently in warmer regions of the world as it did in colder regions [54]. This report is still under review but as with other respiratory viral transmissions, the droplets released during a cough or sneeze are better at staying afloat in colder and dryer air, thereby increasing the chances of transmission [55, 56].

4.6. Low Vitamin D level

Tropical Africa is known to enjoy greater sunshine hours. Exposure to sunlight is known to provide the body's requirement of vitamin D as its insufficiency could affect 50% of the global populace. Vitamin D deficiency (VDD) can lead to hypovitaminosis D pandemic (a risk factor for total mortality) which stems primarily from a person's lifestyle (reduced outdoor movement), and environmental factors like air pollution that reduces exposure to solar radiation, which would influence the dermal production of Vitamin D. Conversely, only a small fraction of our daily consumed foods contain vitamin D. Overall, a lack of this particular vitamin portends negative effects on the immune system and increases the severity of chronic diseases or viral infections. It is recommended that treatment with vitamin D2 or D3 to be administered to deficient patients as vitamin D supplementation is related to declining mortality [57]. Furthermore, it is believed that regular intake of vitamin D supplements may reduce the risks associated with the novel coronavirus infection among the elders who live sedentarily with limited outdoor activities. Recent research also has reported an association between low levels of vitamin D and enhanced transmission of the coronavirus [58]. However, this study is yet to be peer-reviewed and does not explicitly explain whether it is just low levels of vitamin D or there is a possibility of other confounding factors involved. Therefore, there is no scientific evidence to back this claim; the deficiency of Vitamin D may elevate the overall vulnerability to infectious disease by impeding immune functions [59].

5. CONCLUSION

Severe cases of COVID-19 are resulting in breathing changes and hypoxia, leading to unusual respiratory rates that could be an indication of underlying medical issues. Critical cases, though they are rare, are also accompanied by fundamental medical conditions and distinguished by respiratory and organ failure which often require thorough care. Mild cases, being the most predominantly occurring manifestations of the coronavirus infection are mostly characterized by lung infections (inflammation) which are commonly allayed without the need for intensive care. Patients with cardiovascular comorbidities are known to be the most prone to critical or severe instances of the disease, while inflammatory infections are said to be the least threatening co-occurrences. Authors have reported a variety of immune disorders and aberrated chest radiographs as anomalous observations among infected persons. Hence, viral densities of SARS-CoV-2 have been reported to positively correlate to the severity of lung disease. Furthermore, factors such as aging, obesity, immune-deficiency, the asymptomatic nature of the illness as well as gene selectivity and reactivity are reportedly associated to the increased risk of contracting the virus. Similarly, habits such as smoking and alcohol addiction are believed to elevate the risk of contracting COVID-19. Socio-economic components which contribute to the spread of the infection include poverty, illiteracy, ignorance about the disease, popularity of fake/misinformed news and the practical application of unverified scientific claims which has gone agog in social media, further proffering remedial ways of curbing the proliferation of the disease. Based on the foregoing, it is pertinent that co-morbid individuals, especially those who are suffering from cardiovascular ailments should strictly adhere to social distancing rules to prevent them from being infected. While attempting to avoid crowded places by staying indoors the majority of the time, sedentary living should generally be discouraged, but particularly avoided among the aged. This is based on the reported possibility of a strong relationship between outdoor activities, vitamin D supplementation and immune system improvement. Obese individuals may need to reduce weight by engaging in physically activities to improve their breathing rhythm, body mass index and increase their chances of survival in the event of being exposed to COVID-19. In addition, regional governments need to ensure that the public is properly guided with adequate information about the virus, employing effective means of communication with rural dwellers who are the most vulnerable to misinformation.

CONSENT FOR PUBLICATION

Not applicable.

CONFLICT OF INTEREST

The author declares no conflict of interest, financial or otherwise.

ACKNOWLEDGEMENTS

Declared none.

REFERENCES

[1] Kakodkar P, Kaka N, Baig MN. A Comprehensive Literature Review on the Clinical Presentation, and Management of the Pandemic Coronavirus Disease 2019 (COVID-19). Cureus 2020; 12(4): e7560. [http://dx.doi.org/10.7759/cureus.7560] [PMID: 32269893]

[2] Worldometers.info. Coronavirus Cases : Deaths : Worldometer's COVID-19 data.. 2021.http://www.worldometers.info/coronavirus/about/

[3] Meghani SH, Buck HG, Dickson VV, *et al.* The conceptualization and measurement of comorbidity: a review of the interprofessional discourse. Nurs Res Pract 2013; 2013(1): 1-10. [http://dx.doi.org/10.1155/2013/192782] [PMID: 24187618]

[4] Valderas JM, Starfield B, Sibbald B, Salisbury C, Roland M. Defining comorbidity: implications for understanding health and health services. Ann Fam Med 2009; 7(4): 357-63. [http://dx.doi.org/10.1370/afm.983] [PMID: 19597174]

[5] Xie J, Tong Z, Guan X, Du B, Qiu H. Clinical Characteristics of Patients Who Died of Coronavirus Disease 2019 in China. JAMA Netw Open 2020; 3(4): e205619. [http://dx.doi.org/10.1001/jamanetworkopen.2020.5619] [PMID: 32275319]

[6] Langford BJ, So M, Raybardhan S, *et al.* Antibiotic prescribing in patients with COVID-19: rapid review and meta-analysis. Clin Microbiol Infect 2021; 27(4): 520-31. [http://dx.doi.org/10.1016/j.cmi.2020.12.018] [PMID: 33418017]

[7] Tehrani HA, Darnahal M, Vaezi M, Haghighi S. COVID-19 associated thrombotic thrombocytopenic purpura (TTP); A case series and mini-review. Int Immunopharmacol 2021; 93: 107397. [http://dx.doi.org/10.1016/j.intimp.2021.107397] [PMID: 33524803]

[8] Liu Y, Yang Y, Zhang C, *et al.* Clinical and biochemical indexes from 2019-nCoV infected patients linked to viral loads and lung injury. Sci China Life Sci 2020; 63(3): 364-74. [http://dx.doi.org/10.1007/s11427-020-1643-8] [PMID: 32048163]

[9] Wang D, Hu B, Hu C, *et al.* Clinical Characteristics of 138 Hospitalized Patients With 2019 Novel Coronavirus–Infected Pneumonia in Wuhan, China. JAMA 2020; 323(11): 1061-9. [http://dx.doi.org/10.1001/jama.2020.1585] [PMID: 32031570]

[10] Wang L, He W, Yu X, *et al.* Coronavirus disease 2019 in elderly patients: Characteristics and prognostic factors based on 4-week follow-up. J Infect 2020; 80(6): 639-45. [http://dx.doi.org/10.1016/j.jinf.2020.03.019] [PMID: 32240670]

[11] Meng Y, Wu P, Lu W, *et al.* Sex-specific clinical characteristics and prognosis of coronavirus disease-19 infection in Wuhan, China: A retrospective study of 168 severe patients. PLoS Pathog 2020; 16(4): e1008520. [http://dx.doi.org/10.1371/journal.ppat.1008520] [PMID: 32343745]

[12] Xu XW, Wu XX, Jiang XG, *et al.* Clinical findings in a group of patients infected with the 2019 novel coronavirus (SARS-Cov-2) outside of Wuhan, China: retrospective case series. BMJ 2020; 368(January): m606. [http://dx.doi.org/10.1136/bmj.m606] [PMID: 32075786]

[13] Zhang J, Wang X, Jia X, *et al.* Risk factors for disease severity, unimprovement, and mortality in COVID-19 patients in Wuhan, China. Clin Microbiol Infect 2020; 26(6): 767-72. [http://dx.doi.org/10.1016/j.cmi.2020.04.012] [PMID: 32304745]

[14] Guan W, Ni Z, Hu Y, *et al.* Clinical Characteristics of Coronavirus Disease 2019 in China. N Engl J Med 2020; 382(18): 1708-20. [http://dx.doi.org/10.1056/NEJMoa2002032] [PMID: 32109013]

[15] Huang C, Wang Y, Li X, *et al.* Clinical features of patients infected with 2019 novel coronavirus in Wuhan, China. Lancet 2020; 395(10223): 497-506. [http://dx.doi.org/10.1016/S0140-6736(20)30183-5] [PMID: 31986264]

[16] Liu K, Fang YY, Deng Y, *et al.* Clinical characteristics of novel coronavirus cases in tertiary hospitals in Hubei Province. Chin Med J (Engl) 2020; 133(9): 1025-31. [http://dx.doi.org/10.1097/CM9.0000000000000744] [PMID: 32044814]

[17] Özdemir Ö. Coronavirus Disease 2019 (COVID-19): Diagnosis and Management (narrative review).

Erciyes Med J 2020.

[18] Yin Q, Fu Z, Xie J, Yang J, Li F, Zhu W, *et al.* Analysis of Risk Factors of Severe COVID-19 Patients 2020; 1-14.

[19] Lei S, Jiang F, Su W, *et al.* Clinical characteristics and outcomes of patients undergoing surgeries during the incubation period of COVID-19 infection. EClinicalMedicine 2020; 21: 100331. [http://dx.doi.org/10.1016/j.eclinm.2020.100331] [PMID: 32292899]

[20] Tan SC. Clinical and epidemiological characteristics of Coronavirus Disease 2019 (COVID-19) patients. medRxiv 2020. [http://dx.doi.org/10.1101/2020.04.02.20050989]

[21] Zheng J. SARS-coV-2: An emerging coronavirus that causes a global threat. Int J Biol Sci 2020; 16(10): 1678-85. [http://dx.doi.org/10.7150/ijbs.45053] [PMID: 32226285]

[22] Morales L, Oliveros JC, Fernandez-Delgado R, tenOever BR, Enjuanes L, Sola I. SARS-Co--Encoded Small RNAs Contribute to Infection-Associated Lung Pathology. Cell Host Microbe 2017; 21(3): 344-55. [http://dx.doi.org/10.1016/j.chom.2017.01.015] [PMID: 28216251]

[23] Navand SS, Moghadami M, Hosseini P, Nasimzadeh S, Zandi M. Diabetes and coronavirus infections (SARS-CoV, MERS-CoV, and SARS-CoV-2). J Acute Dis 2020; 9(6): 244.http://www.jadweb.org/

[24] Guzik TJ, Mohiddin SA, Dimarco A, *et al.* COVID-19 and the cardiovascular system: implications for risk assessment, diagnosis, and treatment options. Cardiovasc Res 2020; 116(10): 1666-87. [http://dx.doi.org/10.1093/cvr/cvaa106] [PMID: 32352535]

[25] Ryan DH, Ravussin E, Heymsfield S. COVID 19 and the Patient with Obesity – The Editors Speak Out. Obesity (Silver Spring) 2020; 28(5): 847. [http://dx.doi.org/10.1002/oby.22808] [PMID: 32237212]

[26] Wu J, Li W, Shi X, *et al.* Early antiviral treatment contributes to alleviate the severity and improve the prognosis of patients with novel coronavirus disease (COVID-19). J Intern Med 2020; 288(1): 128-38. [http://dx.doi.org/10.1111/joim.13063] [PMID: 32220033]

[27] Cai G, Bossé Y, Xiao F, Kheradmand F, Amos CI. Tobacco smoking increases the lung gene expression of ACE2, the Receptor of SARS-CoV-2. Am J Respir Crit Care Med 2020; 201(12): 1557-9. [http://dx.doi.org/10.1164/rccm.202003-0693LE] [PMID: 32329629]

[28] Smith JC, Sausville EL, Girish V, *et al.* Cigarette Smoke Exposure and Inflammatory Signaling Increase the Expression of the SARS-CoV-2 Receptor ACE2 in the Respiratory Tract. Dev Cell 2020; 53(5): 514-529.e3. [http://dx.doi.org/10.1016/j.devcel.2020.05.012] [PMID: 32425701]

[29] Qiu F, Liang CL, Liu H, *et al.* Impacts of cigarette smoking on immune responsiveness: Up and down or upside down? Oncotarget 2017; 8(1): 268-84. [http://dx.doi.org/10.18632/oncotarget.13613] [PMID: 27902485]

[30] Lang AE, Yakhkind A. Coronavirus Disease 2019 and Smoking. Chest 2020; 158(4): 1770-6. [http://dx.doi.org/10.1016/j.chest.2020.06.013] [PMID: 32561438]

[31] Vardavas C, Nikitara K. COVID-19 and smoking: A systematic review of the evidence. Tob Induc Dis 2020; 18(March): 20. [http://dx.doi.org/10.18332/tid/119324] [PMID: 32206052]

[32] Sarkar D, Jung MK, Wang HJ. Alcohol and the immune system. Alcohol Res 2015; 37(2): 153-5.

[33] Parry CD, Patra J Jr, Rehm J. Alcohol consumption and non-communicable diseases: epidemiology and policy implications. Addiction 2011; 106(10): 1718-24. [http://dx.doi.org/10.1111/j.1360-0443.2011.03605.x] [PMID: 21819471]

[34] Nicholson LB. The immune system. Essays Biochem 2016; 60(3): 275-301. [http://dx.doi.org/10.1042/EBC20160017] [PMID: 27784777]

[35] Jacofsky D, Jacofsky EM, Jacofsky M. Understanding Antibody Testing for COVID-19. J Arthroplasty 2020; 35(7): S74-81. [http://dx.doi.org/10.1016/j.arth.2020.04.055] [PMID: 32389405]

[36] Bretscher PA. On the mechanism determining the TH1/TH2 phenotype of an immune response, and its pertinence to strategies for the prevention, and treatment, of certain infectious diseases. Scand J Immunol 2014; 79(6): 361-76. [http://dx.doi.org/10.1111/sji.12175] [PMID: 24684592]

[37] Andersson U, Ottestad W, Tracey KJ. Extracellular HMGB1: a therapeutic target in severe pulmonary inflammation including COVID-19? Mol Med 2020; 26(1): 42. [http://dx.doi.org/10.1186/s10020-020-00172-4] [PMID: 32380958]

[38] Wong CK, Lam CWK, Wu AKL, *et al.* Plasma inflammatory cytokines and chemokines in severe acute respiratory syndrome. Clin Exp Immunol 2004; 136(1): 95-103. [http://dx.doi.org/10.1111/j.1365-2249.2004.02415.x] [PMID: 15030519]

[39] Mogensen TH. Pathogen recognition and inflammatory signaling in innate immune defenses. Clin Microbiol Rev 2009; 22(2): 240-73. [http://dx.doi.org/10.1128/CMR.00046-08] [PMID: 19366914]

[40] Tay MZ, Poh CM, Rénia L, MacAry PA, Ng LFP. The trinity of COVID-19: immunity, inflammation and intervention. Nat Rev Immunol 2020; 20(6): 363-74. [http://dx.doi.org/10.1038/s41577-020-0311-8] [PMID: 32346093]

[41] Al-Hinai AT, Hassan MO, Simsek M, Al-Barwani H, Bayoumi R. Genotypes and allele frequencies of angiotensin converting enzyme (ACE) insertion/deletion polymorphism among Omanis. J Sci Res Med Sci 2002; 4(1-2): 25-7. [PMID: 24019722]

[42] Delanghe Joris R, Marijn M. Speeckaert MLDB. The host's angiotensin-converting enzyme polymorphism may explain epidemiological findings in COVID-19 infections 2020.

[43] Denis M, Vandeweerd V, Verbeeke R, Laudisoit A, Reid T, Hobbs E, *et al.* 2020.https://rega.kuleuven.be/if/corona_covid-19

[44] Leon DA. Poverty, Inequality and Health. An International Persepective. International Journal of Epidemology 2001; 30.

[45] Zarocostas J. How to fight an infodemic. Lancet 2020; 395(10225): 676. [http://dx.doi.org/10.1016/S0140-6736(20)30461-X] [PMID: 32113495]

[46] Müller O, Krawinkel M. Malnutrition and health in developing countries. CMAJ 2005; 173(3): 279-86. [http://dx.doi.org/10.1503/cmaj.050342] [PMID: 16076825]

[47] McIntyre L, Connor SK, Warren J. Child hunger in Canada: results of the 1994 National Longitudinal Survey of Children and Youth. CMAJ 2000; 163(8): 961-5. [PMID: 11068567]

[48] Marmot M. Social Determinants of Health Inequalities. Lancet 2005;365(9464):1099-104. [http://dx.doi.org/10.1016/S0140-6736(05)71146-6]

[49] Paakkari L, Okan O. COVID-19: health literacy is an underestimated problem. Lancet Public Health 2020; 5(5): e249-50. [http://dx.doi.org/10.1016/S2468-2667(20)30086-4] [PMID: 32302535]

[50] Daniel P. Oran EJT. Prevalence of Asymptomatic SARS-CoV-2 Infection. A Narrative Review. Ann Intermedicine 2020; 173(5): 1-36.

[51] He D, Zhao S, Lin Q, *et al.* The relative transmissibility of asymptomatic COVID-19 infections among close contacts. Int J Infect Dis 2020; 94(April): 145-7.
[http://dx.doi.org/10.1016/j.ijid.2020.04.034] [PMID: 32315808]

[52] Yao Y, Pan J, Liu Z, *et al.* No association of COVID-19 transmission with temperature or UV radiation in Chinese cities. Eur Respir J 2020; 55(5): 2000517.
[http://dx.doi.org/10.1183/13993003.00517-2020] [PMID: 32269084]

[53] Lai AT, Lin IC, Yang YW, Wu MF. Climate change and human health. J Intern Med Taiwan 2012; 23(5): 343-50.

[54] Just J, Puth M-T, Regenold F. Klaus Weckbecker MB. Distinguishing between COVID-19 and the common cold in a primary care setting - comparison of patients with positive and negative SARS-CoV-2 PCR results. medRxiv 2020.

[55] Qasim Bukhari YJ. Will coronavirus pandemic diminish by summer? 2020.

[56] Exploring Physiological Adaptations as Causes of Ethnic Variation in Metabolic Diseases. Anthropology 2013; 01(04): 1-2.

[57] Nair R, Maseeh A, Vitamin D. Vitamin D: The "sunshine" vitamin. J Pharmacol Pharmacother 2012; 3(2): 118-26.
[PMID: 22629085]

[58] Ilie PC, Stefanescu S, Smith L. The role of vitamin D in the prevention of coronavirus disease 2019 infection and mortality. Aging Clin Exp Res 2020; 32(7): 1195-8.
[http://dx.doi.org/10.1007/s40520-020-01570-8] [PMID: 32377965]

[59] Kubala J. 2020.https://www.healthline.com/nutrition/vitamin-d-coronavirus

CHAPTER 3

A Silver Lining for Covid 19: Nutraceuticals and Plant Secondary Metabolites

Neetesh Kumar Jain[1,*] and **Nitu Singh**[1]

[1] *Department of Pharmacology, Oriental College of Pharmacy and Research, Faculty of Pharmacy, Oriental University, Indore, India*

Abstract: There are some confines to the worldwide disease instigated by the novel coronavirus disease 2019 (COVID19), for now, a vaccine or treatment is available. According to SAGE, the Pfizer-BioNTech, COVID-19 mRNA vaccine is safe and effective. Vaccination is not recommended for certain populations due to contraindications, lack of availability, or inadequate data. Individuals with a background of grave allergies, pregnant women, and foreign travellers who are not part of a prioritized group, and children under the age of 16 are all cautioned against getting the vaccine. This necessitates the use of some alternatives that strengthen the immune system. The new therapies and medications provide our bodies with a window duration that aids in the creation of adaptive ion channels. The human immunity system is made up of various body organs and cells that work together with a symphony to defend the host from foreign particles such as viruses, bacteria, fungi, parasites, and so on. To synthesize various types of immune cells, our body needs a broad range of small amounts (vitamins and minerals) and large amounts (carbohydrate, protein, and fat) nutrients. Certain established prehistoric herbs that improve immunity include garlic, basil leaves, and black pepper. The following chapter includes a list of immune-supporting nutraceuticals (such as omega-3 fats, glucans, amino acids, probiotics, vitamins, and minerals) and plant's secondary metabolites, as well as the impression of their supplementation in boosting the body's immunity to make it able to combat COVID-19.

Keywords: Alkaloids, Amino Acids, COVID 19, Coronavirus, Flavonoids, Herbal Extract, Immunity Booster.

1. INTRODUCTION

Coronavirus disease 2019 (COVID-19) is a communicable ailment instigated by the Severe acute respiratory syndrome coronavirus 2 (SARS-CoV-2) [1]. Firstly, it was discovered in Wuhan, China, in December 2019 and has meanwhile blow-

* **Corresponding author Neetesh Kumar Jain**: Department of Pharmacology, Oriental College of Pharmacy and Research, Faculty of Pharmacy, Oriental University, Indore, India; Tel: 91-9479347077;
E-mail: drneetesh@orientaluniversity.in

out internationally, resulting in a pandemic [2]. On average 7.3 million cases stayed registered across 188 countries and territories as of June 10, 2020, resulting in more than 413,000 deaths [3]. As of March 3, 2021, the virus had infected 115 million people worldwide, with 2.54 million people dying as a result of the disease. COVID-19 is a highly contagious, critical illness characterized by Pneumonia and Acute respiratory distress syndrome (ARDS). Severe acute respiratory syndrome coronavirus 2 (SARS-CoV-2), like Middle East respiratory syndrome coronavirus (MERS-CoV) and SARS-CoV-1, comes under the Coronaviridae family and causes the disease. The virus's genome is positive-sense Ribonucleic acid (RNA), which codes for 26 proteins that help the virus survive, replicate as well as propagate in the host. The virus is spread by contact with infected people's aerosol droplets [4]. Coronaviruses are encased viruses with a positive-sense genome of single-stranded RNA (+ssRNA). These viruses are members of the Coronaviridae family and subfamily Coronavirinae, which contaminate birds and mammals through its spike (S) glycoprotein and the virus binds to angiotensin-converting enzyme 2 (ACE2) receptors on cells [5]. S1 and S2 are the two domains of the S protein. S1 binds to the peptidase domain of ACE2, known as the receptor-binding domain (RBD), and membrane fusion is catalyzed by S2, allowing genetic material to be released inside the cells [6]. Individuals' immune status and the occurrence of underlying medical conditions, may influence the beginning of the clinical disease and its progression to a serious level. Dry cough (67 percent), fever (88 percent), exhaustion (38 percent), myalgias (14.9 percent), and dyspnoea (18.7%) are the most common clinical symptoms. Other symptoms comprise headache, sore throat, rhinorrhoea, and gastrointestinal symptoms. Pneumonia is a serious infection indicator. COVID-19 has complicated the pathogenesis that includes the conquest of the host's antiviral and innate immune responses, oxidative stress initiation, and a "cytokine storm" that results in acute lung damage, tissue fibrosis, and pneumonia [7]. Vaccines and other treatments are now currently available, although they have certain limitations. According to the Strategic advisory group of experts on immunization (SAGE), the Pfizer-BioNTech COVID-19 mRNA vaccine is safe and effective. Vaccination is not recommended for certain populations due to contraindications, a lack of availability, or inadequate data. The vaccine is not recommended for people who have a background of serious allergies or who are pregnant, international travellers who are not part of a prioritized group, and children under 16.

COVID-19 is more common in pregnant women than in non-pregnant women, and COVID-19 has been related to an increased risk of preterm birth. The World Health Organisation (WHO), however, does not suggest vaccination of pregnant women at this time due to a lack of evidence.

Vaccination may be given to a breastfeeding woman who is part of a group (*e.g.*, health workers) that has been recommended for vaccination. Breastfeeding should not be interrupted following vaccination, according to the WHO [8].

This necessitates the use of some alternatives that strengthen the immune system. The current therapy and medication are providing our bodies a window of opportunity for the production of adaptive immunity against COVID-19. Nutrition should be on top priority, particularly. Since our immune system is the only thing standing between us and this novel coronavirus-19 (Fig. **1**). In this situation, the WHO issued certain guidelines for obtaining vital nutrients during the pandemic in order to maintain good health [9].

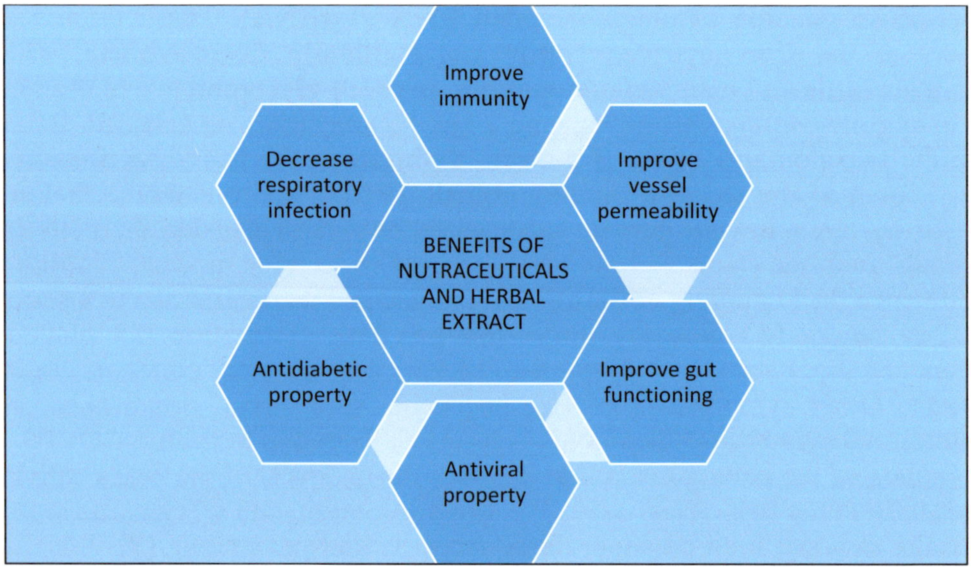

Fig. (1). Diagrammatic representation showing the favourable effects of nutraceuticals and herbal extracts in COVID-19.

Immune cells need adequate energy with macronutrients and micronutrients, serving as co-factors of the growth, articulation, and maintenance of the immunity system. The role of balanced food in the immune system has been extensively recognized, and the effect of various food components on specific aspects of immune function has been extensively researched (Fig. **2**). It is generally accepted that an individual's nutritional status affects their immune ability, which can be taken as a proportion of a satisfactory diet [10].

2. IMMUNITY BOOSTER NUTRIENTS

2.1. Vitamin A

Vitamin A is known as a fat-soluble vitamin. It helps preserve vision, promotes growth and development, and protects the epithelium and mucosal integrity in the human body [11]. It is considered to show a key role in immune function enhancement and immune response control in both cellular and humoral immune responses. Vitamin A supplementation in infants has been shown to increase antibody response after vaccinations such as measles and anti-rabies vaccination (2.1 times) [12]. Because of its important function in enhancing immune ability, vitamin A is also referred to as the "anti-inflammation vitamin". Vitamin A is essential in mucosal epithelial cell integrity and immune capacity. Pre-formed vitamin A (retinol)-liver, egg yolk, butter, milk, and cheese are the animal sources of vitamin A. Fruit and vegetable sources of Pro-vitamin A are carotenoids-orange, flesh fruits (such as sweet potatoes, melon, and mangoes), and green leafy vegetables (spinach, broccoli, carrots, pumpkins, red palm oil). β-carotene is a strong antioxidant agent, by growing disease-fighting cells in the body, it minimizes inflammation and improves immune function [13].

2.2. Vitamin B6

B6 is needed for the stabilization of the blood homocysteine levels, as the rise in homocysteine levels is associated with a high risk of cardiovascular disease. Pyridoxine, pyridoxal, and pyridoxamine are the three moieties present in vitamin B6. All three forms of B6 can be altered to Pyridoxal phosphate (PLP), a coenzyme. Vitamin B6 is included in responses due to its coenzyme structure, and it is safe to say that vitamin B6 is needed for the majority of biological responses in our bodies. Although further study is required to fully comprehend B6's function in immunity. Studies show that Vitamin B6 deficiency affects both humoral and cell-mediated immune responses, effectively disabling immune responses [14]. Vitamin B6 bioavailability: While eating a varied diet, vitamin B6 bioavailability is approximately 75%. Heat destroys vitamin B6, but it stays stable during storage.

Chicken, liver, fish, nuts, chickpeas, maize and whole grain, cereals, and vegetables (especially green leafy vegetables), bananas, potatoes, and other starchy vegetables are all good sources of vitamin B6 [13].

2.3. Vitamin B12

Vitamin B12 is needed for proper red blood cell formation, nerve system function, and Deoxyribonucleic acid (DNA) synthesis. Vitamin B12 acts in combination with Folate and vitamin B6 to support blood homocysteine quantity. Previous literature shows that it is an effective immune modulator for cellular immunity [15]. Vitamin B12, along with folic acid, is important for the immune system's proper functioning. Vitamin B12 deficiency altered immune responses by influencing nucleic acid and protein synthesis, inhibiting immune cell function, and obstructing metabolic processes [16]. Although there is inadequate evidence on vitamin B12 absorption, it is estimated that about 50% of vitamin B12 is consumed by adults having a balanced digestive tract. If there is not sufficient acid in the stomach or a protein known as an intrinsic factor, is not made, inadequate absorption occurs. High heat and long cooking times in traditional cooking methods can cause some vitamin B12 loss. Vitamin B12 comes from a number of sources. It primarily consists of animal sources such as shellfish, liver, and certain fish (herring, sardines, salmon, and trout), as well as milk and milk products [13].

2.4. Vitamin C

This precise nutrient is a chief constituent of the immune system's military. Vitamin C, which is also referred to as ascorbic acid, is a water-soluble vitamin that is important for human health. Humans and a few other species, such as primates and pigs, depend on vitamin C from fruits and vegetables for nutrition (red peppers, oranges, strawberries, broccoli, mangoes and lemons). In medical science, Vitamin C's potential function in preventing and alleviating infection is well known. Vitamin C is necessary for immune function. Anti-inflammatory, immune-modulating, antioxidant, antithrombotic, and antiviral properties are all present. Vitamin C tends to favourably modulate host responses to the COVID-19 pandemic's causal agent, the extremely serious SARS-CoV-2. It aids in the prevention of the common virus. Vitamin C is an important antioxidant that protects the body from the injurious effects of oxidative stress. Vitamin C high-dose intravenous treatment has been shown to dramatically recover indications in patients with critical infections, such as sepsis and ARDS. Vitamin C plays an important part in wound healing and cancer prevention, as it protects cells against the oxidative damage resulting from free radicals. Vitamin C protects against illnesses and uneasiness by promoting the innate and immune systems of different cell capacities. In the case of respiratory tract infections, a Cochrane study found that supplementing members with Vitamin C reduced the frequency of infection significantly [17].

Vitamin C bioavailability: Vitamin C levels in foods are affected by growing environments, season, stage maturity, cookery methods, and storage time earlier to use. Heat and oxygen are the only factors that can degrade vitamin C. The amount of absorption is determined by the amount of food ingested. Vitamin C is consumed to the 70-90 percent. Absorption levels decrease to 50% when intakes reach 1000 mg per day.

Fruits (especially citrus fruits such as lemon, orange, and Indian gooseberry), cabbage, green leafy vegetables, lettuce, tomatoes, potatoes, and liver are all good sources of vitamin C [13].

2.5. Vitamin D

It is a fat-soluble vitamin that helps to control both innate and adaptive immune reactions [18]. By weakening the body's development of pro-inflammatory compounds, Vitamin D supplementation can diminish the risk of viral infections, including respiratory tract diseases. Vitamin D deficiency has been associated with the anticipation of extra infectious diseases such as tuberculosis, hepatitis, and cardiovascular diseases [19]. T regulatory lymphocytes (TRL) are an important line of defense contrary to uncontrolled inflammation and viral contamination in general. TRL levels have been found to be low in many COVID-19 patients, and vitamin D supplementation can help raise them. Vitamin D shortage has been connected to the rise in inflammatory cytokines as well as a higher risk of pneumonia and upper respiratory tract infection. Thrombotic episodes are normal in COVID-19 patients, and vitamin D deficiency is related to a rise in them. Vitamin D deficiencies have been found to be more common in obese and diabetic patients [20]. Supplementing with vitamin D appears to reduce the chances of emerging serious respiratory tract contaminations to varying degrees [21, 22]. In those who were infected, influenza symptoms were less severe and recovery was faster if large doses of vitamin D greater than 1000 IU were administered [23]. Vitamin D comes from a variety of places. Sunlight exposure, in the correct growing condition (not or restricted through water dependent on latitude) and for a sufficient amount of time, plays a critical role in deciding our vitamin D status. Vitamin D is synthesized under the skin through cholesterol as a starting material in the presence of sunlight. Vitamin D is available in two forms: D2 (ergocalciferol) and D3 (cholecalciferol). Natural nutrition sources include oily fish like salmon, herring, and mackerel, red meat, liver, and egg yolk, as well as fortified foods like most fat spread and certain breakfast cereals [13].

2.6. Vitamin E

Vitamin E is a fat-soluble nutrient and is an effective antioxidant with the capacity to affect the immunity system of the host [24]. Vitamin E shortage is believed to affect both humoral as well as cellular immunity. Vitamin E is a remarkable cancer prevention agent that prevents cells from oxidizing free radicals. It has been discovered that it plays a noteworthy role in immune capacity regulation. Even a small amount of vitamin E deficiency has been shown to weaken the immune response and its function in progressing an immune system, which is particularly noticeable in the elderly [25, 26]. Lee and Hang's research have revealed that it plays a particularly protective role against a number of infectious diseases [27]. As stated it is a fat-soluble vitamin, *i.e.* when fat is present in a meal, absorption of this vitamin is increased. Individuals who eat a diet consisting primarily of starchy staples, with irregular consumption of edible oils or other vitamin E-rich vegetables, are at a higher risk of vitamin E deficiency. Edible vegetable oils (such as wheat germ, sunflower, and rapeseed), leafy green vegetables (spinach, chards, *etc.*), almonds, avocados, sunflower seed, mango, and kiwi fruit are all healthy sources of vitamin E [13].

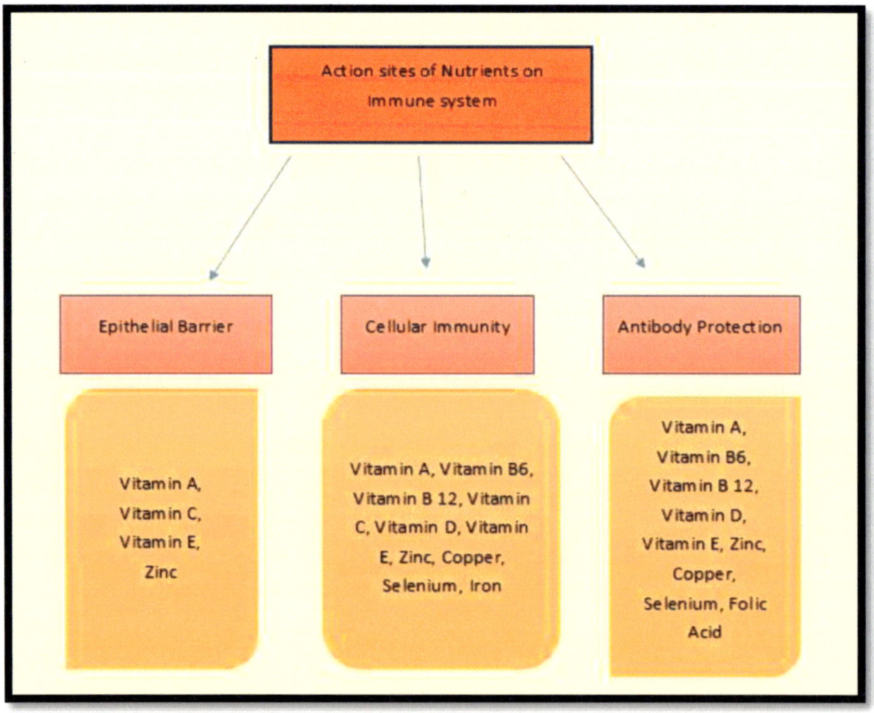

Fig. (2). Diagram representing the role of micronutrients on the immune system.

2.7. Iron

Iron is required for the formation of hemoglobin, which carries oxygen across the body. Iron may also act as a cofactor for enzymes in the oxidation or reduction of responses (*i.e.*, acknowledges or gives electrons). These responses are important for the energy metabolism of cells [28]. Small iron concentrations impair the capacity to mount a proper immune reaction. It is needed for the making and progress of immune cells, especially lymphocytes, which are linked to infection-specific responses. Since many pathogens depend on this basic part, iron appropriation is a significant intrinsic host protection mechanism. Due to this, the body's iron supply is cautiously regulated and attached to proteins such as transferrin and ferritin [29].

Iron bioavailability: The body controls iron absorption, and absorption rates differ depending on the size of a person's iron stores. The absorption of iron is influenced by a number of factors. Vitamin C and animal proteins are two factors that aid in the absorption of organic iron. Phytates, polyphenol, vegetable protein, and calcium are all inhibitors of inorganic iron absorption.

Red meat, seafood, poultry, shellfish, eggs, legumes, grains, and dried fruits are all good sources of iron [13].

2.8. Zinc

Zinc is found in almost every cell in the human body and is an effective addition to growth and enhancement. Muscles, testicles, and bones have the highest concentrations. Zinc levels are tightly regulated by the body. Anxiety and diseases, as a result, cause zinc levels in the blood to drop. Zinc plays an important role in the immune system and wound healing, according to a lot of evidence. Zinc has been shown to affect a variety of immune system components, ranging from the skin's barrier to gene regulation [30]. Both zinc deficiency and excess cause changes in immune cell numbers and behaviours, resulting in increased disease vulnerability and improved resistance to provocative contaminations. Zinc has been shown to reduce oxidative pressure, which has been linked to the prevention of illness [31].

Zinc's bioavailability: Zinc absorption, like iron absorption, is affected by the zinc body pool, with those with low zinc levels being able to absorb zinc more effectively in the gut. Phytate-rich foods cause previously ingested zinc to be lost in the faeces. Zinc absorption can be aided by protein. Meats, shellfish, legumes, whole grains, and fortified cereals are all healthy sources of zinc [13].

2.9. Selenium

It is a mineral that is found in nature. Selenium is an integral constituent of the body's antioxidant system, which protects the body from oxidative stress, which is a natural by-product of metabolic reactions. There is now enough evidence that selenium plays an important role in immune system function [32]. This acknowledges its role in regulating oxidative pressure, redox, and other cell forms in nearly all tissues and cell types, including those involved in innate and adaptive immune responses [33]. Surprisingly, reports have related low selenium levels to the incidence, severity, or disease of certain viral infections. When researching selenium and population, Arthur and colleagues hypothesized that deficiency could contribute to the development of pro-inflammatory compounds, which could increase the risk of illnesses like coronary illness and disease [34].

Selenium bioavailability: Selenium from food sources is very bioavailable.

Seafood, seafood, whole grains, dairy, fruits, and vegetables are all good sources of selenium [13].

2.10. Amino Acids

N-acetyl-cysteine (NAC) is an amino acid that is produced from the naturally occurring amino acid cysteine and is widely administered to patients having respiratory problems such as respiratory tract infections, idiopathic pulmonary fibrosis, and chronic bronchitis [35, 36]. NACs' antioxidant and mucolytic properties have been shown to substantially increase airway role and minimize Chronic obstructive pulmonary disease (COPD) exacerbations [37]. NAC treatment has also been shown to minimize mucin release and prevent Respiratory syncytial virus (RSV) infection in human alveolar epithelial (A549) cells [38]. Sadowska concluded in a previously reported research that NAC may be useful in the treatment of COPD because it promotes mucus clearance, reduces oxidative stress and inflammation [39]. These findings show that NAC has a lot of potential as an adjuvant supplement for COVID-19 patients [40, 41].

2.11. Arginine

Arginine has been shown to work in tandem with virucidal environments including elevated temperatures and acidic pH levels, potentially deactivating enveloped viruses [42]. Tsujimoto *et al.* used an arginine solution to successfully deactivate Herpes simplex virus type 2 (HSV-2) [43]. In the same way, Influenza

A has been shown to be disabled in similar circumstances [44]. Arginine inactivates viruses through a number of mechanisms, including pore formation and membrane destabilization, inhibition of non-structural protein activity, suppression of protein-protein interactions, and aggregation [42]. Arginine interacts with several sites on viral particles, influencing glycoprotein-lipid interactions on the viral envelope [45]. Due to arginine's low cytotoxicity, a previous study showed that an intranasal spray containing an aqueous solution of arginine could be used to prevent influenza A infection *in vivo* [46]. By dropping airway inflammation in lung tissue and varying L-arginine metabolism, arginine has been found to lead to upgraded asthmatic symptoms [47].

2.12. Glutamine (GLN)

With a concentration of around 500-900 mol/l, GLN is one of the most plentiful free amino acids in the human organ system [48]. At therapeutic doses, GLN was found to reduce inflammation by preventing neutrophil enrolment into the airways [49]. The administration of GLN reduced lung tissue damage, lung oedema, cytokine development, and neutrophil recruitment to the lung in a ventilator-induced lung injury (VILI) mouse model, in which mice's lungs are deeply damaged by acid aspiration [50]. Exogenous GLN, according to Oliveira *et al.* can be useful in the treatment of lung cancer, asthma, and ARDS [51]. As a consequence, GLN could be beneficial to COVID-19 patients [52].

3. NUTRACEUTICALS

3.1. Probiotics

Probiotic nutritional supplementation is reported to help patients with respiratory tract infections [53]. Probiotics are living microorganisms that, when ingested, provide health benefits by enhancing or restoring gut flora [54]. It was reported that probiotic strains such as *Lactococcus lactis* W58, *Lactobacillus Brevis* W63, *Enterococcus faecium* W54, *Lactobacillus acidophilus* W22, *Bifidobacterium lactis* W51, and *Bifidobacterium bifidum* W23 reduced the frequency of upper respiratory tract infections (URTIs) in qualified athletes [55]. *Lactobacillus casei* Zhang, a probiotic strain with immunomodulatory, anti-inflammatory, and anti-oxidative properties, has been shown to reduce upper respiratory tract infection symptoms and restore gastrointestinal health in adults and the elderly subjects [56]. Various probiotic strains, including *Lactobacillus gasseri* SBT2055 and *Lactobacillus rhamnosus* CRL1505, have been shown to suppress respiratory syncytial virus infection [57, 58]. Probiotics are important in the treatment of common cold infections, according to a meta-analysis conducted by Kang *et al.*

[59]. The Chinese National Health Commission and the National Administration of Traditional Chinese Medicine recommended probiotic therapy to control coronavirus infection during the COVID-19 pandemic; however, the effectiveness of probiotics in reducing patient mortality in the intensive care unit has, however, to be determined [60]. Jayawardena *et al.* proposed probiotics as a dietary supplement to avoid SARS-CoV-2 infection in susceptible populations [61]. Probiotics can be a useful intervention technique against COVID-19, since they are widely available as dietary supplements and have fewer side effects when used appropriately [62].

3.2. Omega-3 fatty Acids

These are essential fatty acids. Saturated and unsaturated fats are crucial components of the human diet and play an important role in nutrition and health [63]. Fats are the major source of energy, playing a role in cell signalling and responses, and are structurally important as a component of the cell membrane. Patients with respiratory problems such as ARDS, COPD, reduced oxygenation, and pulmonary fibrosis have been confirmed to benefit from omega-3 polyunsaturated fatty acids [64]. They are gaining popularity due to their anticoagulant properties and ability to minimize inflammation [65]. Consumption of omega-3 polyunsaturated fatty acids has been linked to a variety of physiological changes, including lung surfactant development, host-microbial interactions, blood rheology changes, and endogenous eicosanoid production [66]. According to a study, Omega-3 fatty acids can reduce inflammatory problems caused by allergic reactions and asthma [67]. Omega-3 fatty acids have also been shown to inhibit immunoglobulin E synthesis, resulting in decreased airway inflammation and bronchoconstriction in asthma patients [68]. Linday *et al.* discovered that giving children both cod liver oil (which contains eicosapentaenoic acid (EPA) and vitamin A) and a multivitamin-mineral supplement at the same time reduced the mean number of URTI-related medical consultations by a statistically significant (P0.05) amount over time [69]. Overall, omega-3 fatty acids improve the health of patients with upper respiratory tract infection problems and reduce the duration of stay in the hospital for acutely ill patients [70]. Since omega-3 fatty acids have been shown to reduce airway inflammation and bronchoconstriction and have also shown efficacy against viral infections [71], they have the potential to be used against COVID-19 [72].

3.3. β-glucans

β-glucans are active immune cell activators that support the host defence system by activating neutrophils, natural killer cells, and macrophages [73]. β-glucans have been shown to reduce the sensitivity of healthy subjects to upper respiratory tract infections (URTI)s and to minimize the severity of URTIs in infected subjects, in addition to their immunomodulatory impact [74]. Antiviral activity of β-Glucans has also been demonstrated against Herpes simplex viruses (HSV-1) and influenza viruses [75]. More recently, it has been proposed that -glucans can help to reduce COVID-19-related morbidity and mortality [76].

3.4. Secondary Plant Metabolites Against COVID-19 Virus

3.4.1. Alkaloids

Alkaloids are a class of naturally occurring nitrogen-containing compounds with at least one nitrogen heteroatom, usually in the form of a heterocyclic ring with basic properties that produce strong physiological responses [77].

In India [78] and China [79], *Tylophora indica* and *Tylophora ovata* are used as traditional medicines. Tylophorine and tylophorine analogues, which were first isolated from the plant *T. indica*, have been shown to have broad *in vivo* activity against a variety of diseases, including inflammation [80], which is one of the hallmarks of pathogenic coronavirus infection, as well as the ability to inhibit global protein synthesis [81]. Interestingly, tylophorine has also been shown to prevent Hepatitis C virus (HCV) replication. Borreira is Rubiaceae genera that are used to treat and manage diseases including respiratory infections, eye inflammation, malaria, skin diseases, fever, hemorrhage, urinary infections, diarrheal and other digestive disorders, headaches, and gum disease. Borreira's various extracts have been stated to have antioxidant, antimicrobial, anti-inflammatory, antitumor, anti-ulcer, larvicidal, gastrointestinal, and hepatoprotective properties. Bioactive compounds from the plant, such as terpenoids and flavonoids, have been linked to these biological activities, with alkaloids and iridoids as the main active concepts [82]. When tested alongside Remdesivir, lopinavir, and homoharringtonine in their capacity to inhibit SARS-CoV-2 replication *in vitro*, phytochemical screening revealed the presence of an alkaloid called emetine in *B. verticillata* [83]. *A. Emetine* has been reported to have antiviral activity against the SARS-CoV-2 virus in Vero E6 cells with an estimated 50 percent effective concentration of 0.46 uM. Emetine, an antiprotozoal agent, potently inhibits Zika virus (ZIKV) and Ebola virus (EBOV) infection *in vitro* with a low nanomolar half-maximal inhibitory concentration (IC_{50}) and potent activity *in vivo*, according to the findings [84].

3.4.2. Terpenoids

Triterpenes are made up of six isoprene units, with squalene as the template, and are found in a wide range of plant species [85]. They play an imperative role in modulating cellular metabolism, especially sterol biosynthesis, and have antiviral properties [86]. Dammarenediol-II, Dammarenolic acid, Hydroxyl hopanone, Hydroxyl dammarenone-I, Shoreic acid, Ursonic acid, Hydroxyoleanonic lactone, and Eichlerianic acid are among the triterpenes that have been confirmed to have antiviral activity against HSV1 and HSV2 [87]. Terpenoids are important because of their diverse abundance in plants and microorganisms, as well as their low inhibitory concentration (IC50) [88]. Molecular dynamic simulations have also shown that thymoquinone derived from *Nigella sativa* can interfere with SARS-attachment CoV-2's to the heat shock protein A5 (HSPA5) substrate-binding domain b (SBDb) in stress cells, lowering the risk of infection [89]. However, it might be time to switch thymoquinone from bench to clinical trials in the face of the Covid-19 pandemic. Terpenoids were also found to be effective at suppressing the virus protease enzyme activity in the sample [90].

3.4.3. Polyphenols/flavonoids

Polyphenols are the type of phytoconstituents that have great pharmacological significance. Polyphenols are known to boost the immune response of cells to foreign invaders, allowing for cellular accumulation of various types of polyphenols through various receptors. As a consequence, signalling channels are activated, and immune responses are triggered [91]. In an *in-silico* study conducted by Adem *et al.*, natural polyphenols were identified as potent COVID-19 main protease (Mpro) inhibitors. The effectiveness of curative plants based on bioactive phytoconstituents such as flavonoids was assessed against COVID-19 Mpro in this analysis, which was performed by using molecular docking. The COVID-19 virus was docked with 80 different flavonoids, and the results showed that compounds including rutin, apiin, hesperidin, diosmin, and diacetyl curcumin, among others, had an important inhibitory effect on the protease enzyme and may play a role in reducing COVID-19 infection symptoms [92]. With over 5000 different compounds known and listed, flavonoids are an important class of plant secondary metabolites with antiviral therapeutic potential [93]. These secondary metabolites are usually found as glycosides and acyl glycosides in vegetables and fruits and are considered as one of the most abundant polyphenols in the human diet. Flavonoids such as quercetin, naringin, hesperetin, and catechin are found naturally in plants and have been studied for their antiviral activity against a variety of animal viruses like HSV-1, respiratory syncytial virus, parainfluenza virus type 3, and poliovirus type -1 [94]. Flavonoids have been shown to have antiviral activity against *Rous sarcoma*, pseudorabies, adenoviruses, and Sindbis as well as the extreme acute respiratory syndrome coronavirus (SARS-CoV) [95]. They suppress viral infection primarily by inhibiting cellular receptor kinases such as mitogen-activated protein kinase (MAPKs,) serine/threonine-specific protein kinase (Akt), and phosphatidylinositol-4, 5-bisphosphate 3-kinase (PI3-K), which inhibits the cellular signalling cascades [96].

Curcumin, the main curcuminoid in turmeric, has been found to have anti-inflammatory, antioxidant, antimicrobial, hypoglycaemic, wound healing, chemo preventive, chemo-sensitizing, and radio-sensitizing properties and affects multiple signalling pathways [97]. Several curcumin derivatives have been shown to have antiviral properties. Five active curcumin derivatives were found to reduce H1N1-induced neuraminidase activation in H1N1-infected lung epithelial cells in studies using the neuraminidase activation assay [98]. Tetramethyl curcumin and curcumin both inhibit the expression of nucleoproteins. Turmeric derivatives have been found to be effective in the treatment of influenza virus infections by a number of researchers. Monoacetyl curcumin and curcumin both prevented influenza virus infection, but through different pathways. Turmeric has been shown to have antiviral activity against the H5N1 virus (highly pathogenic avian influenza) in Madin–Darby canine kidney (MDCK) cells *in vitro* by interfering with viral haemagglutination (HA) activity [99]. Liquorice root has been used in ancient Egyptian medicine, Indian Ayurvedic medicine, and traditional Chinese medicine for centuries. While the antiviral properties of liquorice root have been identified, scientists discovered that during the SARS epidemic, some groups of people who drank traditional Chinese medicine concoctions containing liquorice root were not infested [100]. Natural products contained in liquorice root include flavonoids such as Glabridin, Liquiritigenin, and Glycyrrhizin, which have antiviral activity against the SARS coronavirus. Triterpenoids contained in liquorice roots, such as glycyrrhizic acid and glycyrrhetinic acid, have been found to be very effective against the SARS coronavirus [101]. The main constituent of *Glycyrrhiza glabra* root is glycyrrhizin, which is high in flavonoids, -sitosterol, hydroxyl coumarins, and glycyrrhetinic acid. Glycyrrhizin has been used to treat a variety of diseases, including bronchitis, gastritis, and jaundice, since ancient times. They have also been shown to have anti-inflammatory and antioxidant properties, as well as the ability to stimulate the production of interferons in the human body. Glycyrrhizin has been found to lessen the ability of SARS-Cov agents to bind to cells, mainly in the primary phases of viral infection. Other studies have also reported Glycyrrhizin's anti-SARS-CoV activity [102]. One report by Jeong and Kim shows that Cellular signalling pathways like Protein kinase C, casein kinase II, and transcription factors such as activator protein 1 and nuclear factor κB are all affected by glycyrrhizin. Furthermore, in macrophages, glycyrrhizin and its aglycone metabolite 18 β glycyrrhetinic acid, upregulate inducible nitrous oxide synthase expression and nitrous oxide output [103]. It was stated that Glycyrrhizin induces nitrous oxide synthase in Vero cells, which suppresses virus replication, according to preliminary findings [104]. According to a report by Booth *et al.* in HIV-1 and chronic hepatitis C virus patients, glycyrrhizin decreased HIV Protein 24 (P24) antigen levels and increased chemokine output. However, after months of glycyrrhizin therapy, some patients experienced uncommon adverse effects such as a rise in blood pressure and hypokalaemia [105].

Garlic is a widely accepted spice that has been shown to be an effective herbal cure utilized for the anticipation and treatment of a number of ailments. Antibacterial, antiviral, anti-protozoal, anti-cancer, anti-fungal, immunomodulatory, anti-inflammatory, hypoglycaemic, and hypocholesterolemic properties have also been recorded [106]. The key ingredient of aqueous extract of garlic or raw garlic suspension is allicin, which has a cholesterol-decreasing effect in both humans and animals. When a garlic bulb is broken, the enzyme alliinase activates alliin, a non-protein amino acid found in whole garlic, resulting in the production of Allicin [107].

Phyto constituents such as Saponin, tannin, carbohydrates, cardio glycoside, alkaloids, flavonoid, phlobatannin, and glycoside have been found in garlic phytochemical screening [108]. Baicalin, a flavone glucuronide derived from the Scutellaria genus, has been shown to have antioxidative and anti-apoptotic properties and has been used to treat diseases such as pulmonary atrial hypertension [109]. Baicalin's anti-SARS-CoV ability was first noticed *in vitro*, with a strong inhibitory effect and significantly lower toxic implications on plant cell lines. As a result of ACE2 enzyme activation, *in-silico* experiments with baicalin resulted in the stimulation of certain compounds that suppressed COVID-19 infection [110].

COVID-19 has been reported to be inhibited by hesperidin, a flavanone glycoside isolated from citrus fruits. The study used the hesperidin-rich citrus peel from waste, which underwent hydrodynamic cavitation-based rapid expansion and acted as an antiviral agent against COVID-19 [111].

4. EMERGING CHALLENGES AND POTENTIAL SOLUTIONS

COVID-19 World pandemic has become the most debated, burning issue in the current scenario and major health concern around the World. Fast mutation in the Covid-19 virus is a major challenge for drug discovery. The use of nutrients, nutraceuticals, and some plant secondary metabolites to modulate and stimulate the immune response in order to reduce the intensity of COVID-19 symptoms are discussed in this chapter. The nutraceuticals are non-toxic and can be used by people of all ages. Furthermore, a combination of natural antiviral elements and immune-stimulating molecules that have been shown to be effective against other upper-respiratory-tract infections may be effective against SARS-CoV2.

A number of strategies and alternative treatments are used by the world populations to control the COVID-19 pandemic and for the prevention. Social distancing, isolation and quarantine, self-protection, restriction of population mobility, disinfection, and standard precautions are some of the major efforts and actions used for controlling the outbreak. However, there are no integrated, confident, and effective control measures for a complete cure, and global control of COVID-19 is challenging.

5. CONCLUSION

The importance of good nutrition in boosting immunity cannot be overstated. The immunity system is the body's defence system against ailment and foreign matters, and it has been a long period of time recognition that some factors, such as stress and diet, have an effect on the immune system's ability. Vitamins and minerals, also known as micronutrients, are supplements that the body requires for the optimum role and are frequently needed in precisely the right quantities. These micronutrients are not created by the body and therefore they must be obtained through food. Food acts as a key component in the successful running of our immunity system, according to various reports. Giving a diet rich in vitamins and minerals promotes the immune system's optimal ability by providing cancer prevention agents to delay cell damage caused by free radicals or by assisting in the recovery of cells damaged by free radicals or by aiding T-cell creation. Despite the lack of data on nutritional components in context to the hazard and harshness of viral diseases such as COVID-19, the importance of nutritious food in immunity has been acknowledged. Vitamin C, vitamin D, and zinc all have immune-boosting and immune-controlling effects, besides they function together to promote aspects of both innate and adaptive immunity, including epithelial obstructions, cell resistance, and antibodies, which make up the three main lines of resistant defence. All things considered, micronutrients are thought to assist in the creation of a balanced immune system. Vitamins A, B, C, D, E, zinc, iron, and selenium are particularly important for boosting immune response, according to a variety of systematic and clinical evidence.

The aim of this chapter is to illustrate the potential of various nutraceuticals and secondary metabolites as COVID-19 treatments. While the solid review of these compounds' ability to tackle the ongoing COVID-19 pandemic has already been published, the new proof is slowly evolving [112]. However, the published experimental report is still suspect, and there are also variations in the data, as some scientific trials failed to produce the desired results [113]. To address these disagreements and explain questions concerning the significance of these phytoconstituents, randomized and controlled trials are needed, taking these issues into account. Aside from a rise in the percentage of cases identified, some patients who have improved from coronavirus are tested positive for the virus again [114]. As a result, medical authentication of compounds that could potentially aid in the battle against the COVID-19 pandemic is critical.

CONSENT FOR PUBLICATION

Not applicable.

CONFLICT OF INTEREST

The author declares no conflict of interest, financial or otherwise.

ACKNOWLEDGEMENTS

Declared none.

REFERENCES

[1] Zhu N, Zhang D, Wang W, *et al.* A novel coronavirus from patients with pneumonia in China 2019. N Engl J Med 2020; 382(8): 727-33.
[http://dx.doi.org/10.1056/NEJMoa2001017] [PMID: 31978945]

[2] Andersen KG, Rambaut A, Lipkin WI, Holmes EC, Garry RF. The proximal origin of SARS-CoV-2. Nat Med 2020; 26(4): 450-2.
[http://dx.doi.org/10.1038/s41591-020-0820-9] [PMID: 32284615]

[3] Contini C, Di Nuzzo M, Barp N, *et al.* The novel zoonotic COVID-19 pandemic: An expected global health concern. J Infect Dev Ctries 2020; 14(3): 254-64.
[http://dx.doi.org/10.3855/jidc.12671] [PMID: 32235085]

[4] Huang C, Wang Y, Li X, *et al.* Clinical features of patients infected with 2019 novel coronavirus in Wuhan, China. Lancet 2020; 395(10223): 497-506.
[http://dx.doi.org/10.1016/S0140-6736(20)30183-5] [PMID: 31986264]

[5] Ahmed SS. The coronavirus disease 2019 (COVID-19): A review. J Adv Med Med Res 2020; 32(4): 1-9.
[http://dx.doi.org/10.9734/jammr/2020/v32i430393]

[6] Grant W, Lahore H, McDonnell S, *et al.* Evidence that vitamin D supplementation could reduce risk of influenza and COVID-19 infections and deaths. Nutrients 2020; 12(4): 988.
[http://dx.doi.org/10.3390/nu12040988] [PMID: 32252338]

[7] Zhang L, Liu Y. Potential interventions for novel coronavirus in China: A systematic review. J Med Virol 2020; 92(5): 479-90.
[http://dx.doi.org/10.1002/jmv.25707] [PMID: 32052466]

[8] https://www.who.int/news-room/feature-stories/detail/who-can-take-the-pfizer-biontech-covid-19--vaccine

[9] Ang L, Lee HW, Kim A, Lee JA, Zhang J, Lee MS. Herbal medicine for treatment of children diagnosed with COVID-19: A review of guidelines. Complement Ther Clin Pract 2020; 39: 101174. [http://dx.doi.org/10.1016/j.ctcp.2020.101174] [PMID: 32379639]

[10] Islam MT, Sarkar C, El-Kersh DM, *et al.* Natural products and their derivatives against coronavirus: A review of the non□clinical and pre□clinical data. Phytother Res 2020; 34(10): 2471-92. [http://dx.doi.org/10.1002/ptr.6700] [PMID: 32248575]

[11] Huang Z, Liu Y, Qi G, Brand D, Zheng S. Role of vitamin A in the immune system. J Clin Med 2018; 7(9): 258. [http://dx.doi.org/10.3390/jcm7090258] [PMID: 30200565]

[12] Siddiqui FQ, Ahmad MM, Kakar F, Akhtar S. The role of vitamin A in en- hancing humoral immunity produced by antirabies vaccine. East Mediterr Health J 2001; 7(4-5): 799-804. [http://dx.doi.org/10.26719/2001.7.4-5.799] [PMID: 15332782]

[13] The Role of Nutrition in the Immune System Part I of II, Sight and Life. Available from https://sightandlife.org/blog/nutritionimmunity/#:~:text=Incorporating%20nutrition&text=Providing%20a%20diet%20high%20in,cell%20production%20(Cohen%202017).

[14] Rail LC, Meydani SN. Vitamin B6 and immune competence. Nutr Rev 1993; 51(8): 217-25. [http://dx.doi.org/10.1111/j.1753-4887.1993.tb03109.x] [PMID: 8302491]

[15] Tamura J, Kubota K, Murakami H, *et al.* Immunomodulation by vitamin B12: augmentation of CD8+ T lymphocytes and natural killer (NK) cell activity in vitamin B12-deficient patients by methyl-B12 treatment. Clin Exp Immunol 2001; 116(1): 28-32. [http://dx.doi.org/10.1046/j.1365-2249.1999.00870.x] [PMID: 10209501]

[16] Mikkelsen K, Apostolopoulos V. Vitamin B12, Folic Acid, and the Immune System. In: Mahmoudi M, Rezaei N, Eds. Nutrition and ImmunitySwitzerland 2019; 103-14. [http://dx.doi.org/10.1007/978-3-030-16073-9_6]

[17] Hemilä H, Louhiala P. Vitamin C for preventing and treating pneumonia. Cochrane Libr 2013; 8(8): CD005532. [http://dx.doi.org/10.1002/14651858.CD005532.pub3] [PMID: 23925826]

[18] Rosen Y, Daich J, Soliman I, Brathwaite E, Shoenfeld Y. Vitamin D and autoimmunity. Scand J Rheumatol 2016; 45(6): 439-47. [http://dx.doi.org/10.3109/03009742.2016.1151072] [PMID: 27191042]

[19] Grant W, Lahore H, McDonnell S, *et al.* Evidence that vitamin D supplementation could reduce risk of influenza and COVID-19 infections and deaths. Nutrients 2020; 12(4): 988. [http://dx.doi.org/10.3390/nu12040988]

[20] Weir EK, Thenappan T, Bhargava M, Chen Y. Does vitamin D deficiency increase the severity of COVID-19? Clin Med (Lond) 2020; 20(4): e107-8. [http://dx.doi.org/10.7861/clinmed.2020-0301] [PMID: 32503801]

[21] Chung C, Silwal P, Kim I, Modlin RL, Jo EK. Vitamin D-cathelicidin axis: at the crossroads between protective immunity and pathological inflammation during infection. Immune Netw 2020; 20(2): e12. [http://dx.doi.org/10.4110/in.2020.20.e12] [PMID: 32395364]

[22] Charan J, Goyal J, Saxena D, Yadav P. Vitamin D for prevention of respiratory tract infections: A systematic review and meta-analysis. J Pharmacol Pharmacother 2012; 3(4): 300-3. [http://dx.doi.org/10.4103/0976-500X.103685] [PMID: 23326099]

[23] Vuichard Gysin D, Dao D, Gysin CM, Lytvyn L, Loeb M. Effect of vitamin D3 supplementation on respiratory tract infections in healthy individuals: A systematic review and meta-analysis of randomized controlled trials. PLoS One 2016; 11(9): e0162996. [http://dx.doi.org/10.1371/journal.pone.0162996] [PMID: 27631625]

[24] James IE, Ajanwachukwu N, Animoke OP, *et al.* Immune response, anaemia and oxidative stress in

Trypanosoma brucei infected rats fed vitamin E supplemented diet. Antiinfect Agents 2016; 14(1): 28-37.
[http://dx.doi.org/10.2174/2211352514011603021221153]

[25] Moriguchi S, Muraga M. Vitamin E and immunity. Vitam Horm 2000; 59: 305-36.
[http://dx.doi.org/10.1016/S0083-6729(00)59011-6] [PMID: 10714244]

[26] Meydani SN, Han SN, Wu D. Vitamin E and immune response in the aged: molecular mechanisms and clinical implications. Immunol Rev 2005; 205(1): 269-84.
[http://dx.doi.org/10.1111/j.0105-2896.2005.00274.x] [PMID: 15882360]

[27] Lee G, Han S. The Role of Vitamin E in Immunity. Nutrients 2018; 10(11): 1614.
[http://dx.doi.org/10.3390/nu10111614] [PMID: 30388871]

[28] Soyano A, Gómez M. Role of iron in immunity and its relation with infections. Arch Latinoam Nutr 1999; 49(3) (Suppl. 2): 40S-6S.
[PMID: 10971835]

[29] Cassat JE, Skaar EP. Iron in infection and immunity. Cell Host Microbe 2013; 13(5): 509-19.
[http://dx.doi.org/10.1016/j.chom.2013.04.010] [PMID: 23684303]

[30] Shankar AH, Prasad AS. Zinc and immune function: the biological basis of altered resistance to infection. Am J Clin Nutr 1998; 68(2) (Suppl.): 447S-63S.
[http://dx.doi.org/10.1093/ajcn/68.2.447S] [PMID: 9701160]

[31] Maywald M, Wessels I, Rink L. Zinc Signals and Immunity. Int J Mol Sci 2017; 18(10): 2222.
[http://dx.doi.org/10.3390/ijms18102222] [PMID: 29064429]

[32] Hoffmann PR, Berry MJ. The influence of selenium on immune responses. Mol Nutr Food Res 2008; 52(11): 1273-80.
[http://dx.doi.org/10.1002/mnfr.200700330] [PMID: 18384097]

[33] Broome CS, McArdle F, Kyle JAM, *et al.* An increase in selenium intake improves immune function and poliovirus handling in adults with marginal selenium status. Am J Clin Nutr 2004; 80(1): 154-62.
[http://dx.doi.org/10.1093/ajcn/80.1.154] [PMID: 15213043]

[34] Arthur JR, McKenzie RC, Beckett GJ. Selenium in the immune system. J Nutr 2003; 133(5) (Suppl. 1): 1457S-9S.
[http://dx.doi.org/10.1093/jn/133.5.1457S] [PMID: 12730442]

[35] Homma S, Azuma A, Taniguchi H, *et al.* Efficacy of inhaled N-acetylcysteine monotherapy in patients with early stage idiopathic pulmonary fibrosis. Respirology 2012; 17(3): 467-77.
[http://dx.doi.org/10.1111/j.1440-1843.2012.02132.x] [PMID: 22257422]

[36] Blasi F, Page C, Rossolini GM, *et al.* The effect of N -acetylcysteine on biofilms: Implications for the treatment of respiratory tract infections. Respir Med 2016; 117: 190-7.
[http://dx.doi.org/10.1016/j.rmed.2016.06.015] [PMID: 27492531]

[37] Santus P, Corsico A, Solidoro P, Braido F, Di Marco F, Scichilone N. Oxidative stress and respiratory system: pharmacological and clinical reappraisal of N-acetylcysteine. COPD 2014; 11(6): 705-17.
[http://dx.doi.org/10.3109/15412555.2014.898040] [PMID: 24787454]

[38] Mata M, Sarrion I, Armengot M, *et al.* Respiratory syncytial virus inhibits ciliagenesis in differentiated normal human bronchial epithelial cells: effectiveness of N-acetylcysteine. PLoS One 2012; 7(10): e48037.
[http://dx.doi.org/10.1371/journal.pone.0048037] [PMID: 23118923]

[39] Sadowska AM. *N* -Acetylcysteine mucolysis in the management of chronic obstructive pulmonary disease. Ther Adv Respir Dis 2012; 6(3): 127-35.
[http://dx.doi.org/10.1177/1753465812437563] [PMID: 22361928]

[40] Andreou A, Trantza S, Filippou D, Sipsas N, Tsiodras S. COVID-19: The potential role of copper and N-acetylcysteine (NAC) in a combination of candidate antiviral treatments against SARS-CoV-2. In

Vivo 2020; 34(3 suppl) (Suppl.): 1567-88.
[http://dx.doi.org/10.21873/invivo.11946] [PMID: 32503814]

[41] Jaiswal N, Bhatnagar M, Shah H. N-acetycysteine: A potential therapeutic agent in COVID-19 infection. Med Hypotheses 2020; 144: : 110133.. https://www.ncbi.nlm.nih.gov/pmc/articles/PMC7380211/
[http://dx.doi.org/10.1016/j.mehy.2020.110133] [PMID: 32758904]

[42] Meingast C, Heldt CL. Arginine-enveloped virus inactivation and potential mechanisms. Biotechnol Prog 2020; 36(2): 50-60.
[http://dx.doi.org/10.1002/btpr.2931]

[43] Tsujimoto K, Uozaki M, Ikeda K, *et al.* Solvent-induced virus inactivation by acidic arginine solution. Int J Mol Med 2010; 25(3): 433-7.
[PMID: 20127049]

[44] Yamasaki H, Tsujimoto K, Koyama AH, Ejima D, Arakawa T. Arginine facilitates inactivation of enveloped viruses. J Pharm Sci 2008; 97(8): 3067-73.
[http://dx.doi.org/10.1002/jps.21224] [PMID: 18186461]

[45] Ikeda K, Yamasaki H, Minami S, *et al.* Arginine inactivates human herpesvirus 2 and inhibits genital herpesvirus infection. Int J Mol Med 2012; 30(6): 1307-12.
[http://dx.doi.org/10.3892/ijmm.2012.1149] [PMID: 23042569]

[46] Ikeda K, Yamasaki H, Suzuki Y, Koyama AH, Arakawa T. Novel strategy with acidic arginine solution for the treatment of influenza A virus infection. Exp Ther Med 2010; 1(2): 251-6.
[http://dx.doi.org/10.3892/etm_00000039] [PMID: 22993536]

[47] Zhang R, Kubo M, Murakami I, *et al.* L-Arginine administration attenuates airway inflammation by altering L-arginine metabolism in an NC/Nga mouse model of asthma. J Clin Biochem Nutr 2015; 56(3): 201-7.
[http://dx.doi.org/10.3164/jcbn.14-140] [PMID: 26060350]

[48] Pierre JF, Heneghan AF, Lawson CM, Wischmeyer PE, Kozar RA, Kudsk KA. Pharmaconutrition Review. JPEN J Parenter Enteral Nutr 2013; 37(5_suppl) (Suppl.): 51S-65S.
[http://dx.doi.org/10.1177/0148607113493326] [PMID: 24009249]

[49] Lee CH, Kim HK, Kim JM, *et al.* Glutamine suppresses airway neutrophilia by blocking cytosolic phospholipase A(2) *via* an induction of MAPK phosphatase-1. J Immunol 2012; 189(11): 5139-46.
[http://dx.doi.org/10.4049/jimmunol.1201599] [PMID: 23109722]

[50] Lai CC, Liu WL, Chen CM. Glutamine attenuates acute lung injury caused by acid aspiration. Nutrients 2014; 6(8): 3101-16.
[http://dx.doi.org/10.3390/nu6083101] [PMID: 25100435]

[51] Oliveira G, de Abreu M, Pelosi P, Rocco P. Exogenous glutamine in respiratory diseases: Myth or reality? Nutrients 2016; 8(2): 76.
[http://dx.doi.org/10.3390/nu8020076] [PMID: 26861387]

[52] Romano L, Bilotta F, Dauri M, *et al.* Short Report - Medical nutrition therapy for critically ill patients with COVID-19. Eur Rev Med Pharmacol Sci 2020; 24(7): 4035-9.
[PMID: 32329880]

[53] West NP, Horn PL, Pyne DB, *et al.* Probiotic supplementation for respiratory and gastrointestinal illness symptoms in healthy physically active individuals. Clin Nutr 2014; 33(4): 581-7.
[http://dx.doi.org/10.1016/j.clnu.2013.10.002] [PMID: 24268677]

[54] Maldonado J, Cañabate F, Sempere L, *et al.* Human milk probiotic Lactobacillus fermentum CECT5716 reduces the incidence of gastrointestinal and upper respiratory tract infections in infants. J Pediatr Gastroenterol Nutr 2012; 54(1): 55-61.
[http://dx.doi.org/10.1097/MPG.0b013e3182333f18] [PMID: 21873895]

[55] Strasser B, Geiger D, Schauer M, *et al.* Probiotic supplements beneficially affect tryptophan-

kynurenine metabolism and reduce the incidence of upper respiratory tract infections in trained athletes: A randomized, double-blinded, placebo-controlled trial. Nutrients 2016; 8(11): 752. [http://dx.doi.org/10.3390/nu8110752] [PMID: 27886064]

[56] Hor YY, Lew LC, Lau ASY, *et al.* Probiotic Lactobacillus casei Zhang (LCZ) alleviates respiratory, gastrointestinal & RBC abnormality *via* immuno-modulatory, anti-inflammatory & anti-oxidative actions. J Funct Foods 2018; 44(5): 235-45. [http://dx.doi.org/10.1016/j.jff.2018.03.017]

[57] Kitazawa H, Villena J. Modulation of respiratory TLR3-anti-viral response by probiotic microorganisms: Lessons learned from Lactobacillus rhamnosus CRL1505. Front Immunol 2014; 5: 201. [http://dx.doi.org/10.3389/fimmu.2014.00201] [PMID: 24860569]

[58] Eguchi K, Fujitani N, Nakagawa H, Miyazaki T. Prevention of respiratory syncytial virus infection with probiotic lactic acid bacterium Lactobacillus gasseri SBT2055. Sci Rep 2019; 9(1): 4812. [http://dx.doi.org/10.1038/s41598-019-39602-7] [PMID: 30886158]

[59] Kang EJ, Kim SY, Hwang IH, Ji YJ. The effect of probiotics on prevention of common cold: a meta-analysis of randomized controlled trial studies. Korean J Fam Med 2013; 34(1): 2-10. [http://dx.doi.org/10.4082/kjfm.2013.34.1.2] [PMID: 23372900]

[60] Mak JWY, Chan FKL, Ng SC. Probiotics and COVID-19: one size does not fit all. Lancet Gastroenterol Hepatol 2020; 5(7): 644-5. [http://dx.doi.org/10.1016/S2468-1253(20)30122-9] [PMID: 32339473]

[61] Jayawardena R, Sooriyaarachchi P, Chourdakis M, Jeewandara C, Ranasinghe P. Enhancing immunity in viral infections, with special emphasis on COVID-19: A review. Diabetes Metab Syndr 2020; 14(4): 367-82. [http://dx.doi.org/10.1016/j.dsx.2020.04.015] [PMID: 32334392]

[62] Baud D, Dimopoulou Agri V, Gibson GR, Reid G, Giannoni E. Using probiotics to flatten the curve of coronavirus disease COVID-2019 pandemic. Front Public Health 2020; 8: 186. [http://dx.doi.org/10.3389/fpubh.2020.00186] [PMID: 32574290]

[63] Ibarguren M, López DJ, Escribá PV. The effect of natural and synthetic fatty acids on membrane structure, microdomain organization, cellular functions and human health. Biochim Biophys Acta Biomembr 2014; 1838(6): 1518-28. [http://dx.doi.org/10.1016/j.bbamem.2013.12.021] [PMID: 24388951]

[64] Lemoine S CM, Brigham EP, Woo H, *et al.* Omega-3 fatty acid intake and prevalent respiratory symptoms among U.S. adults with COPD. BMC Pulm Med 2019; 119(97): 0852-4.

[65] Whyand T, Hurst JR, Beckles M, Caplin ME. Pollution and respiratory disease: can diet or supplements help? A review. Respir Res 2018; 19(1): 79. [http://dx.doi.org/10.1186/s12931-018-0785-0] [PMID: 29716592]

[66] Knapp HR. Omega-3 fatty acids in respiratory diseases: a review. J Am Coll Nutr 1995; 14(1): 18-23. [http://dx.doi.org/10.1080/07315724.1995.10718468] [PMID: 7706605]

[67] Miyata J, Arita M. Role of omega-3 fatty acids and their metabolites in asthma and allergic diseases. Allergol Int 2015; 64(1): 27-34. [http://dx.doi.org/10.1016/j.alit.2014.08.003] [PMID: 25572556]

[68] Yates CM, Calder PC, Ed Rainger G. Pharmacology and therapeutics of omega-3 polyunsaturated fatty acids in chronic inflammatory disease. Pharmacol Ther 2014; 141(3): 272-82. [http://dx.doi.org/10.1016/j.pharmthera.2013.10.010] [PMID: 24201219]

[69] Linday LA, Tapia-Mendoza J, Shindledecker RD, Dolitsky JN. Effect of daily cod liver oil and a multivitamin-mineral supplement with selenium on upper respiratory tract pediatric visits by young, inner-city, Latino children: randomized pediatric sites. Ann Otol Rhinol Laryngol 2004; 113(11): 891-901.

[http://dx.doi.org/10.1177/000348940411301108] [PMID: 15562899]

[70] Langlois PL, D'Aragon F, Hardy G, Manzanares W. Omega-3 polyunsaturated fatty acids in critically ill patients with acute respiratory distress syndrome: A systematic review and meta-analysis. Nutrition 2019; 61: 84-92.
[http://dx.doi.org/10.1016/j.nut.2018.10.026] [PMID: 30703574]

[71] Calder PC. Omega-3 fatty acids and inflammatory processes: from molecules to man. Biochem Soc Trans 2017; 45(5): 1105-15.
[http://dx.doi.org/10.1042/BST20160474] [PMID: 28900017]

[72] Imai Y. Role of omega-3 PUFA-derived mediators, the protectins, in influenza virus infection. Biochim Biophys Acta Mol Cell Biol Lipids 2015; 1851(4): 496-502.
[http://dx.doi.org/10.1016/j.bbalip.2015.01.006] [PMID: 25617737]

[73] Elena DMC, Calder PC, Roche HM. β-1,3/1,6-glucans and immunity: State of the art and future directions. Mol Nutr Food Res. Jan; 2021; 65(1): e1901071.

[74] Dharsono T, Rudnicka K, Wilhelm M, Schoen C. Effects of yeast (1,3)-(1,6)-beta-glucan on severity of upper respiratory tract infections: a double-blind, randomized, placebo-controlled study in healthy subjects. J Am Coll Nutr 2019; 38(1): 40-50.
[http://dx.doi.org/10.1080/07315724.2018.1478339] [PMID: 30198828]

[75] Murphy EA, Davis JM, Brown AS, *et al.* Benefits of oat β-glucan on respiratory infection following exercise stress: role of lung macrophages. Am J Physiol Regul Integr Comp Physiol 2008; 294(5): R1593-9.
[http://dx.doi.org/10.1152/ajpregu.00562.2007] [PMID: 18353878]

[76] Geller A, Yan J. Could the induction of trained immunity by β-Glucan serve as a defense against COVID-19.Front Immunol.2020 Jul; 11:1782

[77] Sanders JM, Monogue ML, Jodlowski TZ, Cutrell JB. Pharmacologic treatments for coronavirus disease 2019 (COVID-19): A review. JAMA 2020; 323(18): 1824-36.
[http://dx.doi.org/10.1001/jama.2020.6019] [PMID: 32282022]

[78] Raina V, Raina S. The responsiveness of leukocyte adenyl cyclase to tylophorine in asthmatic subjects. Biochem Biophys Res Commun 1980; 94(4): 1074-7.
[http://dx.doi.org/10.1016/0006-291X(80)90528-8] [PMID: 7396949]

[79] You X, Pan M, Gao W, *et al.* Effects of a novel tylophorine analog on collagen-induced arthritis through inhibition of the innate immune response. Arthritis Rheum 2006; 54(3): 877-86.
[http://dx.doi.org/10.1002/art.21640] [PMID: 16508970]

[80] Yang CW, Chuang TH, Wu PL, Huang WH, Lee SJ. Anti-inflammatory effects of 7-methoxycryptopleurine and structure–activity relations of phenanthroindolizidines and phenanthroquinolizidines. Biochem Biophys Res Commun 2007; 354(4): 942-8.
[http://dx.doi.org/10.1016/j.bbrc.2007.01.065] [PMID: 17274949]

[81] Wang Y, Lee S, Ha Y, *et al.* Tylophorine Analogs Allosterically Regulates Heat Shock Cognate Protein 70 And Inhibits Hepatitis C Virus Replication. Sci Rep 2017; 7(1): 10037.
[http://dx.doi.org/10.1038/s41598-017-08815-z] [PMID: 28855547]

[82] Conserva L, Ferreira J Jr. Borreria and Spermacoce species (Rubiaceae): A review of their ethnomedicinal properties, chemical constituents, and biological activities. Pharmacogn Rev 2012; 6(11): 46-55.
[http://dx.doi.org/10.4103/0973-7847.95866] [PMID: 22654404]

[83] Moreira EA. Identification of emetine in some Borreria species (paper chromatography). Trib Farm (Curitiba) 1964; 32: 9-30.

[84] Yang S, Xu M, Lee EM, *et al.* Emetine inhibits Zika and Ebola virus infections through two molecular mechanisms: inhibiting viral replication and decreasing viral entry. Cell Discov 2018; 4(1): 31.
[http://dx.doi.org/10.1038/s41421-018-0034-1] [PMID: 29872540]

[85] Banno N, Akihisa T, Tokuda H, *et al.* Anti-inflammatory and antitumor-promoting effects of the triterpene acids from the leaves of *Eriobotrya japonica.* Biol Pharm Bull 2005; 28(10): 1995-9. [http://dx.doi.org/10.1248/bpb.28.1995] [PMID: 16204964]

[86] Malinowska M, Sikora E, Ogonowski J. Production of triterpenoids with cell and tissue cultures. Acta Biochim Pol 2013; 60(4): 731-5. [PMID: 24432325]

[87] Poehland BL, Carté BK, Francis TA, Hyland LJ, Allaudeen HS, Troupe N. *In vitro* antiviral activity of dammar resin triterpenoids. J Nat Prod 1987; 50(4): 706-13. [http://dx.doi.org/10.1021/np50052a022] [PMID: 2828553]

[88] Augustin JM, Kuzina V, Andersen SB, Bak S. Molecular activities, biosynthesis and evolution of triterpenoid saponins. Phytochemistry 2011; 72(6): 435-57. [http://dx.doi.org/10.1016/j.phytochem.2011.01.015] [PMID: 21333312]

[89] Elfiky AA. Natural products may interfere with SARS-CoV-2 attachment to the host cell. J Biomol Struct Dyn 2020; (May): 1-10. [http://dx.doi.org/10.1080/07391102.2020.1761881] [PMID: 32340551]

[89] Ahmad A, Rehman MU, Alkharfy KM. An alternative approach to minimize the risk of coronavirus (Covid-19) and similar infections. Eur Rev Med Pharmacol Sci 2020; 24(7): 4030-4. [PMID: 32329879]

[91] Ding S, Jiang H, Fang J. Regulation of immune function by polyphenols. J. Immunol. Res. Apr 2018; 0614-20.

[92] Adem S, Eyupoglu V, Sarfraz I, Rasul A, Ali M. Identification of potent COVID-19 main protease (Mpro) inhibitors from natural polyphenols: an *in silico* strategy unveils a hope against CORONA. Preprints 2020.

[93] Ververidis F, Trantas E, Douglas C, Vollmer G, Kretzschmar G, Panopoulos N. Biotechnology of flavonoids and other phenylpropanoid-derived natural products. Part I: Chemical diversity, impacts on plant biology and human health. Biotechnol J 2007; 2(10): 1214-34. [http://dx.doi.org/10.1002/biot.200700084] [PMID: 17935117]

[94] Kaul TN, Middleton E Jr, Ogra PL. Antiviral effect of flavonoids on human viruses. J Med Virol 1985; 15(1): 71-9. [http://dx.doi.org/10.1002/jmv.1890150110] [PMID: 2981979]

[95] Yi L, Li Z, Yuan K, *et al.* Small molecules blocking the entry of severe acute respiratory syndrome coronavirus into host cells. J Virol 2004; 78(20): 11334-9. [http://dx.doi.org/10.1128/JVI.78.20.11334-11339.2004] [PMID: 15452254]

[96] Villa TG, Feijoo-Siota L, Rama JLR, Ageitos JM. Antivirals against animal viruses. Biochem Pharmacol 2017; 133: 97-116. [http://dx.doi.org/10.1016/j.bcp.2016.09.029] [PMID: 27697545]

[97] Gopinath H, Karthikeyan K. Turmeric: A condiment, cosmetic and cure. Indian J Dermatol Venereol Leprol 2018; 84(1): 16-21. [http://dx.doi.org/10.4103/ijdvl.IJDVL_1143_16] [PMID: 29243674]

[98] Lai Y, Yan Y, Liao S, *et al.* 3D-quantitative structure–activity relationship and antiviral effects of curcumin derivatives as potent inhibitors of influenza H1N1 neuraminidase. Arch Pharm Res 2020; 43(5): 489-502. [http://dx.doi.org/10.1007/s12272-020-01230-5] [PMID: 32248350]

[99] Richart SM, Li YL, Mizushina Y, *et al.* Synergic effect of curcumin and its structural analogue (Monoacetylcurcumin) on anti-influenza virus infection. Yao Wu Shi Pin Fen Xi 2018; 26(3): 1015-23. [PMID: 29976394]

[100] Jakkapong W. Further Research into the Phytochemicals Contained in Licorice Root Might Yield A Treatment for the New Coronavirus Strain in China. Thailand Medical News 2020; 3: 39-60.

[101] Hoever G, Baltina L, Michaelis M, *et al.* Antiviral activity of glycyrrhizic acid derivatives against SARS-coronavirus. J Med Chem 2005; 48(4): 1256-9. [http://dx.doi.org/10.1021/jm0493008] [PMID: 15715493]

[102] Feng Yeh C, Chih Wang K, Chai Chiang L, Shieh DE, Hong Yen M, San Chang J. Water extract of licorice had anti-viral activity against human respiratory syncytial virus in human respiratory tract cell lines. J Ethnopharmacol 2013; 148(2): 466-73. [http://dx.doi.org/10.1016/j.jep.2013.04.040] [PMID: 23643542]

[103] Jeong HG, Kim JY. Induction of inducible nitric oxide synthase expression by 18β-glycyrrhetinic acid in macrophages. FEBS Lett 2002; 513(2-3): 208-12. [http://dx.doi.org/10.1016/S0014-5793(02)02311-6] [PMID: 11904152]

[104] Cinatl J, Morgenstern B, Bauer G, Chandra P, Rabenau H, Doerr HW. Glycyrrhizin, an active component of liquorice roots, and replication of SARS-associated coronavirus. Lancet 2003; 361(9374): 2045-6. [http://dx.doi.org/10.1016/S0140-6736(03)13615-X] [PMID: 12814717]

[105] Booth CM, Matukas LM, Tomlinson GA, *et al.* Clinical features and short-term outcomes of 144 patients with SARS in the greater Toronto area. JAMA 2003; 289(21): 2801-9. [http://dx.doi.org/10.1001/jama.289.21.JOC30885] [PMID: 12734147]

[106] Rehman Z, Munir MT. Effect of garlic on the health and performance of broilers. Open Access J Vet 2015; 3(1): 32-9.

[107] Chowdhury SR Sr, Chowdhury SD, Smith TK. Effects of dietary garlic on cholesterol metabolism in laying hens. Poult Sci 2002; 81(12): 1856-62. [http://dx.doi.org/10.1093/ps/81.12.1856] [PMID: 12512577]

[108] Pavni K, Esha B, Neha J, Tushar A. Phytochemical screening of developing garlic and effect of its aqueous extracts on viability of cardiac cell line. J Pharm Res 2011; 4(3): 902-4.

[109] Chen F, Chan KH, Jiang Y, *et al. In vitro* susceptibility of 10 clinical isolates of SARS coronavirus to selected antiviral compounds. J Clin Virol 2004; 31(1): 69-75. [http://dx.doi.org/10.1016/j.jcv.2004.03.003] [PMID: 15288617]

[110] Liu H, Ye F, Sun Q, *et al.* Scutellaria baicalensis extract and baicalein inhibit replication of SARS-CoV-2 and its 3C-like protease *in vitro*. 2020; 21: 34-50.

[111] Meneguzzo F, Ciriminna R, Zabini F, Pagliaro M. Hydrodynamic cavitation- based rapid expansion of hesperidin-rich products from waste citrus peel as a po- tential tool against COVID-19. Preprints 2020.

[112] Umesh KD, Kundu D, Selvaraj C, Singh SK, Dubey VK. Identification of new anti-nCoV drug chemical compounds from Indian spices exploiting SARS-CoV-2 main protease as target. J Biomol Struct Dyn 2020; (May): 1-9. [http://dx.doi.org/10.1080/07391102.2020.1763202] [PMID: 32362243]

[113] Paintsil E, Cheng YC. Antiviral agents. Encyclopedia Microbiology 2019; 176-225.

[114] Xing Y, Mo P, Xiao Y, Zhao O, Zhang Y, Wang F. Post-discharge surveillance and positive virus detection in two medical staff recovered from coronavirus disease 2019 (COVID-19), China, January to February 2020. Euro Surveill 2020; 25(10): 2000191. [http://dx.doi.org/10.2807/1560-7917.ES.2020.25.10.2000191] [PMID: 32183934]

CHAPTER 4

Risk Factors of Covid-19 Enhancing Transmission and Aggravating Patient's Condition

Vishal Trivedi[1,*], **Vinod Nautiyal**[2] and **Retno Widyowati**[3]

[1] *Department of Pharmacy, Madhav University, Abu Road, Pindwara, Rajasthan, India*

[2] *Department of Pharmaceutical Sciences, Gurukul Kangri University Haridwar, Uttarakhand, India*

[3] *Department of Pharmaceutical Science, Faculty of Pharmacy, Universitas Airlangga, Surabaya, 60115, Indonesia*

Abstract: For the last couple of years, novel coronavirus or SAR-CoV-2 is a severe threat to the world. This new strain of coronavirus emerged on 14th December 2020 and has been infecting many parts of the population around the world to date. These viral spikes will bind with the angiotensin-converting enzymes. Many clinical studies conducted have highlighted the association between cardiovascular diseases and COVID-19. It increases the mortality rate, the risk of injury in myocardial, acute coronary syndromes and thromboembolism. COVID-19 has produced some risk factors such as age and gender as well as comorbidities. Coronavirus may pose several challenges for oncology patients. Among cancer patients, severe respiratory and systemic infection are evident specifically among immunosuppressed and ageing patients. Cancer is said to worsen due to COVID-19 as it is linked with inflammatory burst and lymphopenia. This study has discussed the risk factors in COVID-19 transmission, factors that can aggravate it and clinical interactions between the cardiovascular system. Furthermore, several drugs that have been administered against the virus are believed to affect the patients.

Keywords: Cancer and Cardiovascular System, COVID-19, Risk Factors.

1. INTRODUCTION

The world had ceased in December 2019 when the coronavirus outbreak was first reported inWuhan, China . From then on, the virus had spread all over the world and it was declared a global pandemic, affecting every country in the world. The effects of the virus remain unprecedented on public health [1, 2] as well as on

* **Corresponding author Vishal Trivedi:** Department of Pharmacy, Madhav University, Abu Road, Pindwara, Rajasthan, India; Email: vishaltrivediqa@gmail.com

social and economic activity. The number of confirmed cases around the world would increase every day over the last six months. Till date, there is no definitive prevention available across the world. The genus *beta coronavirus* mainly caused COVID-19 [3, 4]. The other two corona viruses which also have contributed to the pandemic are Severe Acute Respiratory Coronavirus(SAR-COV) and the Middle East Respiratory Syndrome Coronavirus (MERS-CoV). COVID-19 causes a respiratory infection as well as signs of pneumonia and acute respiratory distress syndrome (ADRS) [5, 6]. This is because these coronaviruses would trigger cytokine storm like tumour necrosis, IL-β, and IL-6 which are released by the immune system,causing multiorgan failure. Furthermore,coagulations in a substantial proportionamong patients could take place, leading to thromboembolic events. The biological features have shown that 79.6% of genomic sequence is identified [7, 8]. It shows that boththe diseases may enter the body in the same way, triggering the binding of viral spike (S) protein to ACE2 in the host cells. Clinical data shows that the susceptibility to COVID-19 is strongly associatedwith cardiovascular diseases. This has been observed amonga large number of COVID-19 patients which further increases the comorbidities and mortality rate of the virus [9, 10]. Moreover, it can alsoresult in myocardial injury, acute coronary syndrome and thromboembolism. Children too have been affected by COVID-19. The virus could cause hyper inflammatory shock, cardiac dysfunction and coronary vessel abnormalities [11, 12]. There is a bidirectional interaction between the cardiovascular system and COVID-19. This mechanism however is quite elusive. *De novo* cardiovascular damage is developed in a subclinical disorder. ACE2 surface protein plays the most important role in the virus entry. Pathophysiology plays the most crucial role in the development of therapies. There have been around 45 to 50 million of coronavirus cases and the virus has killed around 1.2 to 1.5 million people. Symptoms such as dyspnea, respiratory frequency, blood oxygen saturation and arterial pressure are commonly seen among patients. Some cases of COVID-19 have also shown respiratory failure and mechanism ventilation, shocks as well as coagulopathy. The utilisation of immunopathology is helpful for the identification of clinician patients with a higher risk as they may require prioritised treatment due to rapid progression and adverse outcomes of the infection [13 - 15]. As for demographic risk factors, age, sex and ethnicity complication play animportant role as well. Some risk factors would lead to the high risk of the illness. This is because, the cellular serine protease (TMPRSS2) is formed, thus implicating cancer and viral infections. The ACE2 is expressed in alveolar cells type 2. It is also present in the endothelial and smooth muscle cells. The paucisymptomatic and asymptomatic forms depicta substantial fraction in COVID-19 with comorbidities [16, 17] which include acute respiratory failure, cytokine storm, prothrombotic, organ dysfunction and even death. Cancer patients are more susceptible to COVID-19 as compared to non-cancer patients as a risk factor like cancer has shown high prevalence to the virus. However, as respiratory failure is one of the symptoms of the virus, hematology lung and breast cancers are considered more vulnerable than other types of cancer. In lieu to this, the virus has mostly affected lung cancer patients. There are several countries thathave reported cases of cancer patients with traces of small amount of COVID-19 infection. Cancer prevalence however is not associated with infection risk as lung carcinoma is visible in CT scan manifestations. Other than that, gender, obesity and congestive heart failure are also considered as risk factors. In relation to COVID-19, race and ethnicity are believed to be risk factors as well with Hispanic and Black people are the most affected race and ethnicities with this disease [18 - 20]. Furthermore, the Veneto region has shown higher number of cases and death related to COVID-19. The comorbidities also would increase for former smokers and chemotherapy patients. At older age, the haematological malignancies are the diagnosis of myeloid leukaemia and the cell neo plasma associated would be worsening [21, 22]. Metastatic or stage IV carcinomas patients are more likely to contract COVID-19. Moreover, the severity of the cancer treatment also contributes to the risk factor of the virus. In a multivariant analysis of patients, age and immune inhibitor treatment are also associated with COVID-19 in which about 2.5% of patients are tested positive. It remains unclear whether cancer has higher risk factor or cancer associated risks depend on the demography. However, it is apparent that the combination of cancer diagnosis and COVID-19 is far more dangerous with a risk of death.

2. COVID-19 BIOLOGY (GENOME, GENE AND PROTEINS)

Genomic sequencing is done to understand the characteristics of COVID-19which would help to evaluate the structure of the viral protein. Coronavirus belongs to the family of single-stranded RNA envelope which is highly pathogenic for human beings. MERS-COV is considered as highly pathogenic coronavirus as well. Both of these coronaviruses are originated from bats. SARS-COV-2 is 80% similar to SARS-CoV and 97% similar to bat coronavirus (RaTG13). Based on the homology of genomic sequences, the biological features are also similar to SARS-CoV. ACE2 receptor is utilised by both infections to enter into the host cells. Meanwhile, dipeptidyl peptidaseis used in MERS-CoV. The crown like structure formed contains four types of proteins which are known as (S) spike, (E) envelope, (M) membrane and a (N) nucleocapsid [25 - 27] (Fig. **1**). N proteins would surround the viral genome in a positive sense. Both genome and mRNA would function as a single-stranded rRNA. α, β, γ and δ are shown in coronavirus in which α and β coronaviruses have infected humans. *Beta coronavirus* is the genus from SARS-CoV, MERS-CoV and SARS-CoV-2. The genome sequence of COVID-19 is approximately 30kb in length, consisting of ORFs (open reading frames) which can be utilised for the encoding of 24-27 genes. Pp1a and pp1ab polyproteins would be able to encode 5' terminal of two third of genome which would cleave 16 non-structural proteins such as RNA-dependent and RNA polymerase. On the other hand, the 3′-terminal would encode the structural proteins [S, E, M and N] of one-third of genome. The S protein is employed for virus attachment and pathogenesis. In both coronaviruses, the S protein would trigger the ACE2 into the host cells. Therefore, the S proteins and ACE2 are utilised for the development of vaccines. They are also used in the formation of antibiotics and antiviral drugs [28 - 30].The S proteins are similar in both of the coronaviruses infections in which they consist of73% to 76% of whole proteins and 50% to 60% of receptor binding domain and motif. However, the S proteins which are also present in the new coronavirus differ than the old ones as they show high binding affinity to ACE2 receptors. This can be seen through cryogenic electron microscopy thus making it clear that they have higher affinity in COVID-19. High binding is also related to high severity and transmissibility of COVID-19. 12 nucleosides are inserted into the S proteins to form novel furin cleavage sites [31 - 33] which are not originated from COVID-19 and their functions remain unknown. However, they have been detected in influenza virus and Newcastle disease. They are also used to expand the cells and tissue tropism in COVID-19 and affect the multi-organ [34] (Fig. **2**).

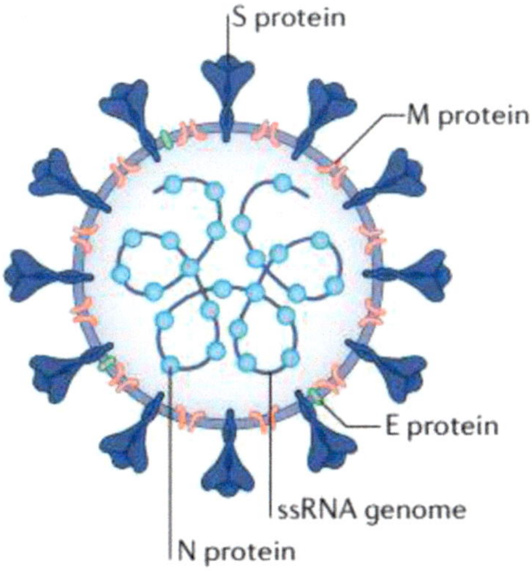

Fig. (1). Structure of coronavirus.

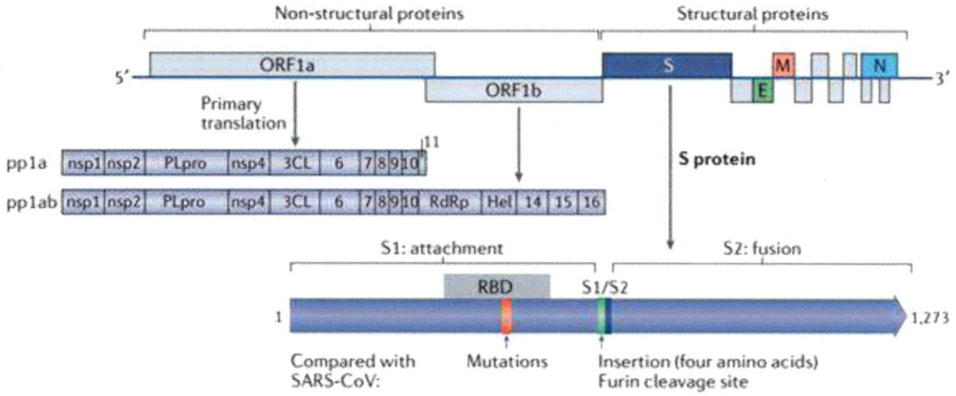

Fig. (2). Genome sequence of coronavirus.

2.1. Virus Life Cycle

S protein is bound to the ACE2 receptor on the surface of the host cell, in which the S1 subunit of the receptor binding domain is responsible for the binding to ACE2. On the other hand, the TMPRSS2 transmembrane serine protease would bind to the S protein. It facilitates the binding of viral membrane thus assisting the virus to enter into the cytoplasm. The epithelial cells in both respiratory tracts used for the expression of ACE2 and TMPRSS2 have predominated the entry of the virus and affected the respiratory tissues. The endosomal entry pathway is utilised by the ACE2 virus and translocated the S protein and endosomes for the cysteine proteases cathepsins B and L [35, 36]. After the completion of this step, the virus would release into the cytoplasm. Lysosomotropic agents and cathepsin inhibitors would block the endosomal entry pathway and predominate the pathway of coronavirus. Polyproteins of ORFs would be translated into the cytoplasm and help to cleave the viral proteases into RdRP. As for the replication of genomic RNA into viral RdRP, the fur structural protein are translated into the endoplasmic reticulum and Golgi complex. With that, the exocytosis would release the new viral particles of genomic RNA. Viral life cycle is described for the potential targets, S proteins, membrane fusion and endocytosis as well as the replication of RNA [37, 38] (Fig. **3**).

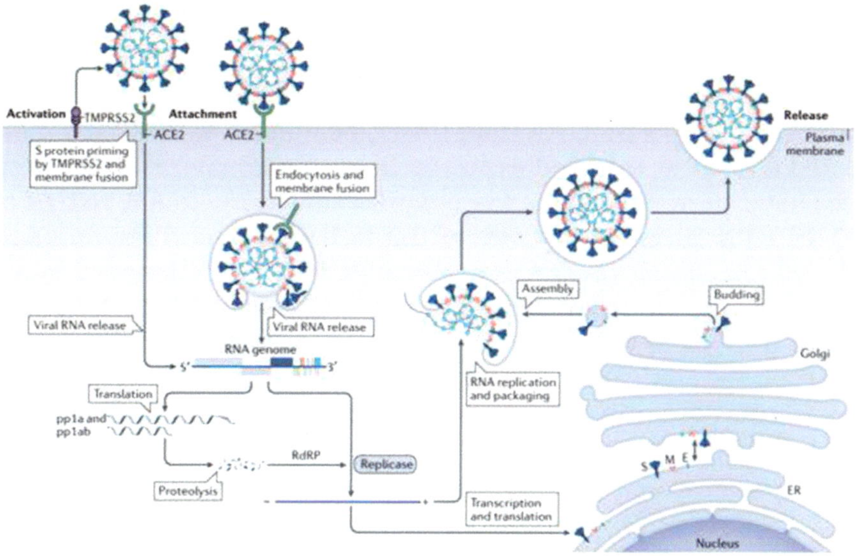

Fig. (3). Virus Life Cycle.

3. FACTORS OF DEMOGRAPHIC

3.1. Age and Gender

The demographic factors are responsible for the cohorts and higher disease severity as healthy and median age peoplerequire more intensive care. 20% to 50% of COVID-19 patients have shown to be severe and critically ill due to the virus. In addition, male gender is believed to be more affected than female gender as ventilation is mostly done among male patients. Moreover, patients between the age of 30 to 60 are more likely to succumb to death when the symptoms occur. Therefore, biological evaluation is the optimal predictor for the disease severity with the pheno age markers [39, 40].

3.2. Ethnicity

Currently, South Asians have the highest number of death due to COVID-19 at 10,930. In New York City, the hospitalisation of Hispanic patients is higher but it is not due to the illness and mortality. The diseases severity has increased among African Americans in South California. However, COVID-19 infections are higher among white people who are associated with diabetes. Low number of death recorded among black ethnicity is said to be due to the end stage of kidney diseases. Therefore, the situations demonstrated in the United Stateshaveshown that race is not considered as the identified risk of death in COVID-19.

4. FACTORS RELATED TO OCCUPATIONS

There are several factors related to occupations that would make them more susceptible to the infection. As front liners, healthcare workers are more likely to be affected with viral load and exposure time of coronavirus. Data from different countries have shown that healthcare workers have 3% to 4% risk of contracting COVID-19 with the mortality rate of 0.2 to 0.3%. According to a survey done, about 10,000 health workers were affected in Wuhan, China 1.5% of them had succumbed to the virus. Furthermore, approximately 20% to 30% of health workers in Italy have been affected by COVID-19 due to exposure to the viral particles from the clinical lung function test done with the patients. The risk factor would increase depending on the severity of COVID-19 and specific activities engaged [43, 44].

4.1. Smoking

Generally, smokers would have high expression of airway epithelial cells therefore, they are more likely to produce infections. Smoking increases the severity and mortality of COVID-19. According to the results of meta-analysis, the majority of COVID-19 patients have smoking history. Current and former smokers can increase the risk of COVID-19 thereby increasing the rate of in-hospital morality, progression of disease and mechanical ventilation. This type of study however does not clarify whether COVID-19 might really affect smokers or smoking related disease such as coronary heart disease and COPD [45, 46].

5. COMPLICATION IN COVID-19

5.1. Acute Kidney Injury (AKI)

Kidney injury is more frequently observed among COVID-19 patients. In the early stage of COVID-19, 0.6% to 30% of patients are affected from AKI. In New York City, 48% of patients are hospitalized due to AKI. Proteinuria and haematuria provide 85% and 82% of risk among COVID-19 patients, respectively. They are done by RRT (renal replacement therapy). AKI and intubated patients would require 87% and 24% of RRT (Fig. **4**). ICU patients of AKI have higher risk than non-AKI patients. Due to this, the identification of soluble urokinase plasminogen activator receptors is done for the immunological risk factor of AKI. The increase observed in suPAR, a biomarker of AKI and COVID-19 [47, 48] would increase the incidence of patient level.

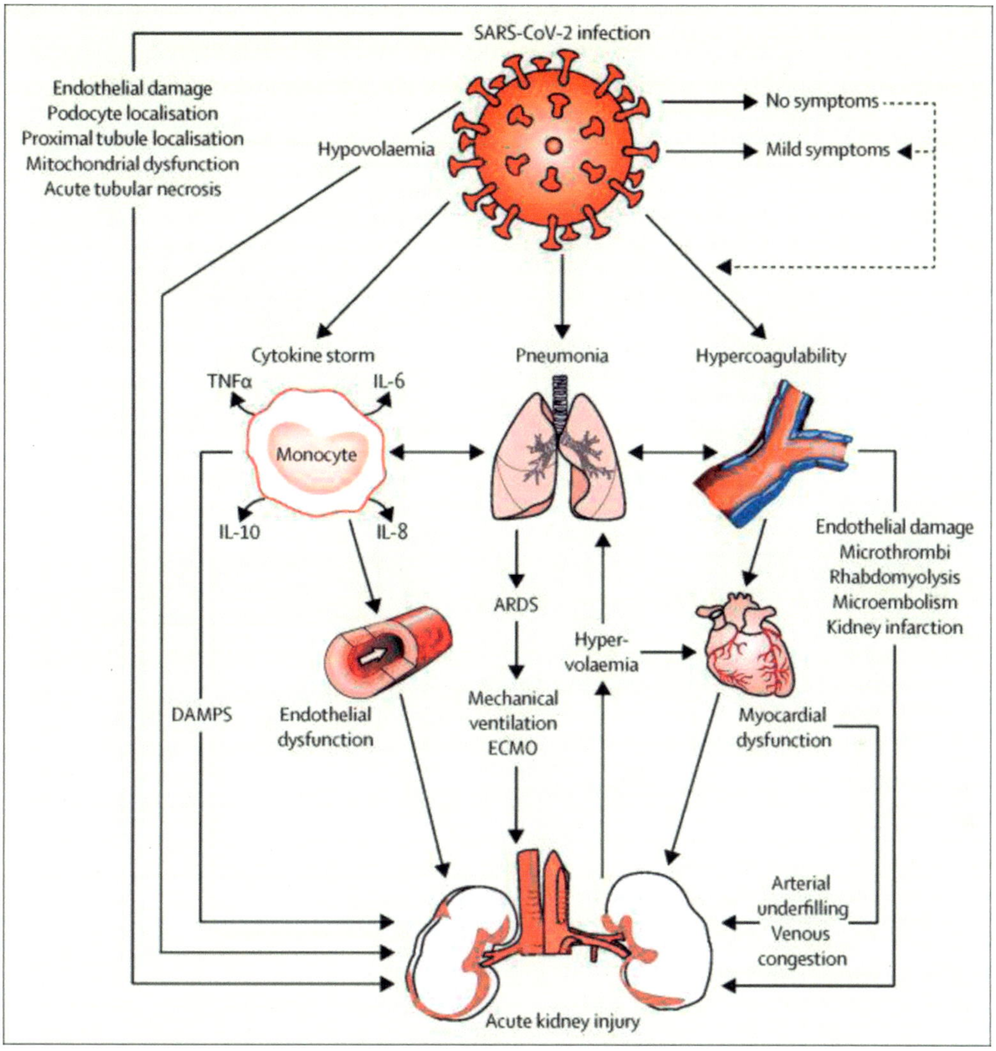

Fig. (4). Acute kidney injury.

5.2. Coagulation Disorders

These conditions would occur when the thrombosis level increases, platelet count decreases, prothrombin time and APTT (activated thromboplastin and fibrinogen) level increase. PT level would increase among severe and critically ill patients. Not only that, the fibrinogen level is also high among severe patients. In some cases, the level is high and demonstrates APTT> 37s which indicates cardiovascular complications (Fig. **5**). In prophylactic and anticoagulant therapy, the bleeding association is higher than normal patients. However, patients with congenital coagulation would have fewer COVID-19 symptoms [49, 50].

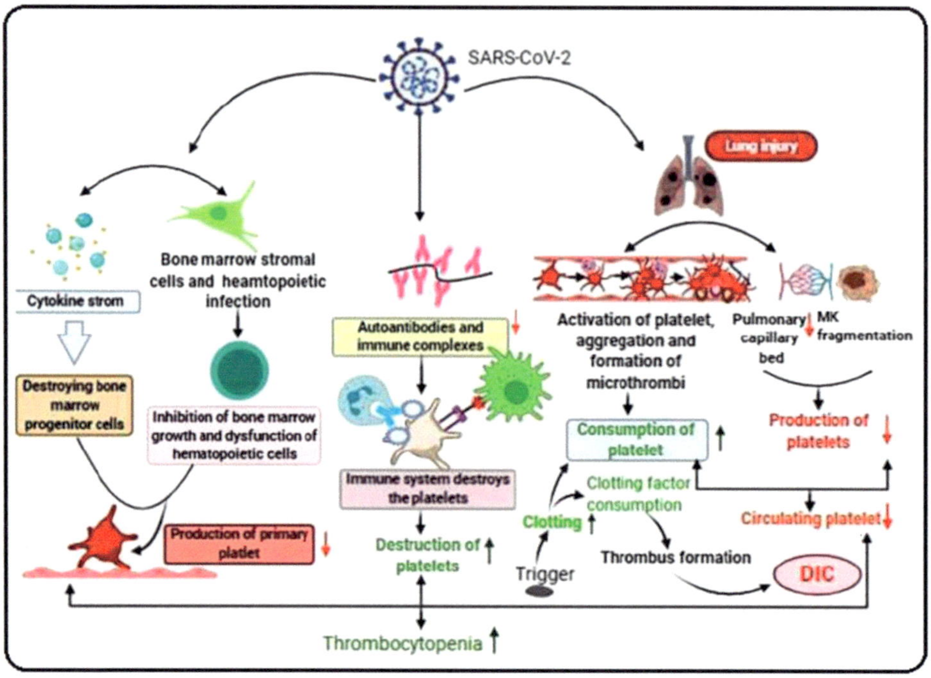

Fig. (5). COVID-19 Effect on Coagulation Disorders.

5.3. Thromboembolism

Other than pneumonia, thromboembolism has a higher risk among COVID-19 patients as the virus can affect the endothelial cells and disrupt the cell membrane. Based on routine clinical care conducted in New York City, 16% to 17% of patients are thrombotic. The number however might be higher as computed tomography pulmonary angiography images have indicated higher incidence of 25%. Furthermore, severe and critical cases of COVID-19 also would have thromboembolism complications. This is due to the inflammation developed by strong cytokines. In mild cases of thromboembolism, the PE and microthrombi of small vessels and microvasculature have hypoxemia and poorer clinical outcome. Development of other diseases such as myocardial infarction and ischemia stroke is also possible among severe and critical cases [51, 52].

5.4. Anticoagulants

A prophylactic and anticoagulant therapy is often utilised among patients with a higher risk of COVID-19 as it helps to reduce the mortality and intubation rates. Among severe COVID-19patients, the need for mechanical ventilation would decrease due to the therapeutic enoxaparin which improves the gas exchange (Fig. **6**). The utilisation of anticoagulant therapy also would reduce the mortality of COVID-19 [53, 54].

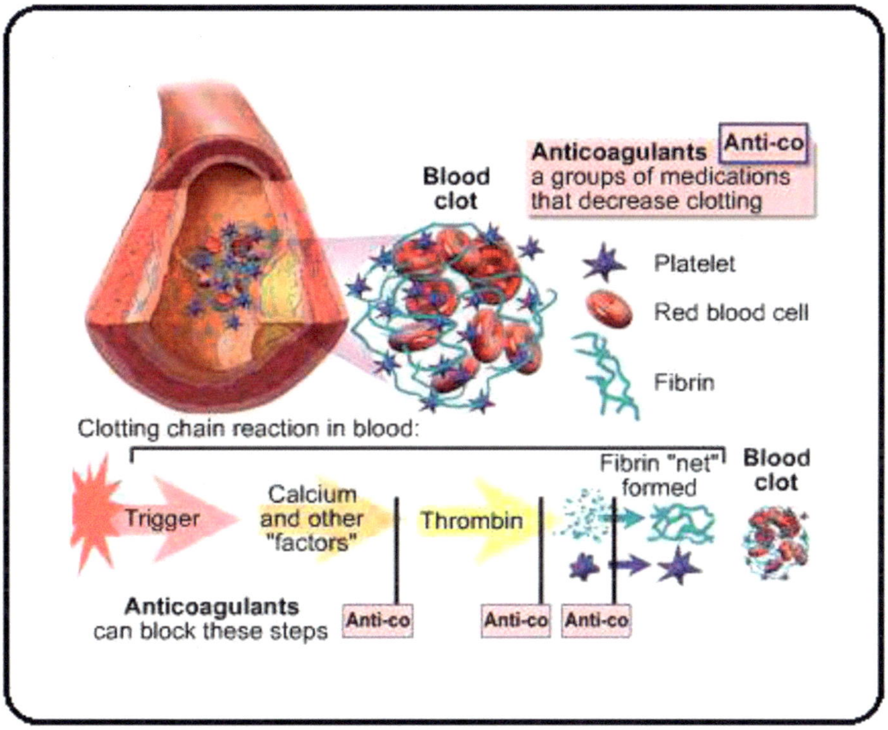

Fig (6). Anticoagulants.

6. RISK FACTOR OF CANCER AND COVID-19

This is to elucidate the relationship between COVID-19 and cancer, specifically the pre-existing of pro-inflammatory and immunosuppression conditions.

6.1. Inflammation and Immune-Senescence

Aging is the most important factor for both COVID-19 and cancer in which immunosenescence and inflammation are related to it. In immunosenescence, the immune system may decline its function and produce insufficient maladaptive respond to vaccination. It also increases debilitating autoimmune diseases. The marker of inflammation is associated with T cells which are lower among COVID-19 patients. The disease severity shows high amount of plasma blasts such as ferritin, D dimers and C reactive. Coronavirus shows cell polarization and gene expression which could be related to inflammation and senescence cellular. Aging association to dysregulation of immune responses would depict the vulnerability to COVID-19 as aging may compromise the antigens and infectious agents. Therefore, older people are more vulnerable due to the low development of immune responses and vaccination. The T cells are also crossed against seasonal coronavirus and it would reduce the risk of antibiotic resistance [55 - 57] (Fig. **7**).

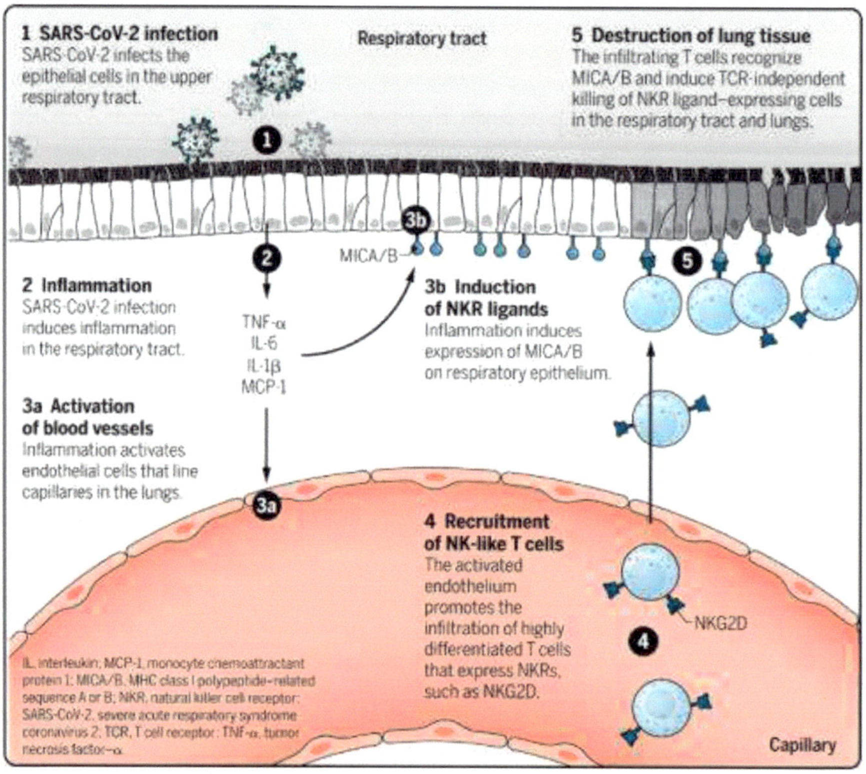

Fig. (7). Inflammation And Immune-Senescence.

6.2. Metabolic Syndrome

There is a strong relationship between cancer and type 2 diabetes. It is believed that people who are morbidly obese have higher risk of contracting COVID-19 and its complications. Diabetic patients too are at risk of contracting COVID-19. This is because insulin hormone would metabolise the tumour and increase obesity . Treatment is very important to mitigate the severity of diseases. Furin and cellular protease would facilitate the viral entry to the S1 and S2 domain of spike protein. Chemotaxis and intercellular killing of microbes are due to the impairment of immunity for the activation of type 1 T cell. Hyperinflammatory response also can be seen in diabetic patients, depending on TH1/ cytotoxic immune responses. The intestinal barrier would facilitate the virus entry and depict the metabolic syndrome. Furthermore, the bacterial translocation would facilitate the epithelial cells and infect the intestinal. Pro-angiogenic and immunosuppression would occur among cancer patients [58 - 60] (Fig. **8**).

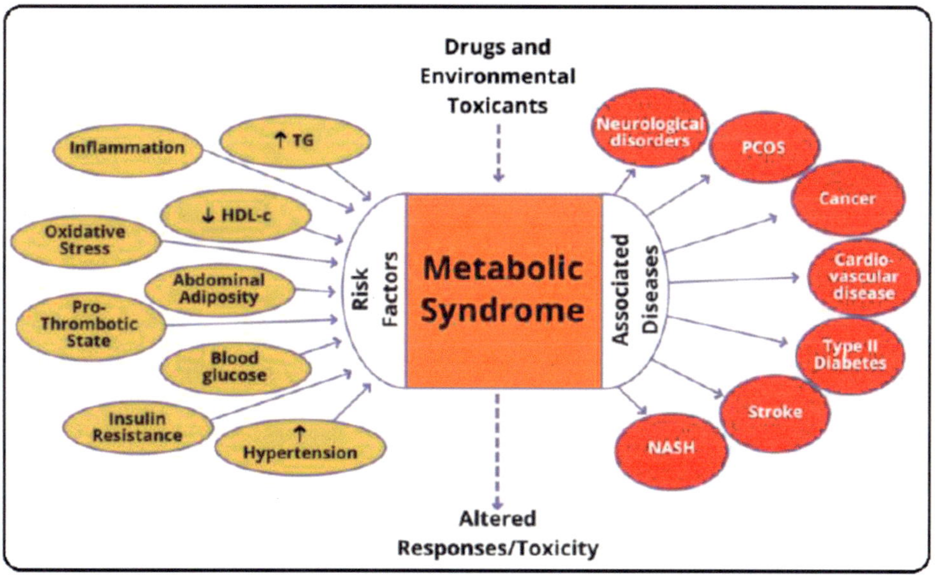

Fig. (8). Metabolic Syndrome.

6.3. Immunosuppression, Interferon and Neutrophilia

Lymphocytes are able to control the progression and therapeutic response of cancer. Class I and class II of histocompatibility complex would express the immunodominant epitopes to form or recognize T lymphocytes cells of CD4+ and

CD8+. The viral infection of immunosuppressive CD4+ lymphopenia can cause pancreatic cancer, breast cancer and others. It mostly affects CD4+ T cells which would increase the risk of febrile neutropenia. However, it has side effects similar to chemotherapy and steroids. Nonetheless, it also helps in the diagnosis of cancer and treatment. Lymphocyte counts however can decrease with radiotherapy. The neutrophile to lymphocyte ratio is marked elevated which decreases the lymphocyte counts. It is a poor prognostic marker and has a blockage of cell death protein among COVID-19 patients (Fig. **9**) [61, 62].

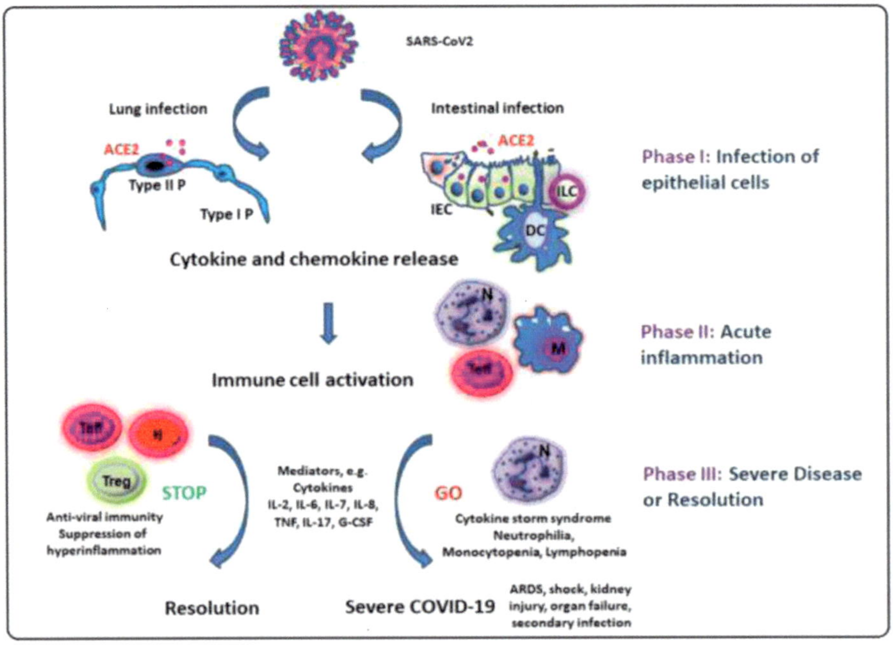

Fig.(9). Immunosuppression, Interferon and Neutrophilia.

6.4. Relationships Between Cancer and Covid-19 Susceptibility or Therapies

There are many factors that contribute to cancer development such as aging and metabolic syndrome. In some patients, the metastatic dissemination and ECOG performance are hampered. The severity of COVID-19 infection can be enhanced due to genotoxic chemotherapies. Aging and obesity also can decline the functions of immune system andincrease the risk of contracting COVID-19 (Fig. **10**) [63, 64].

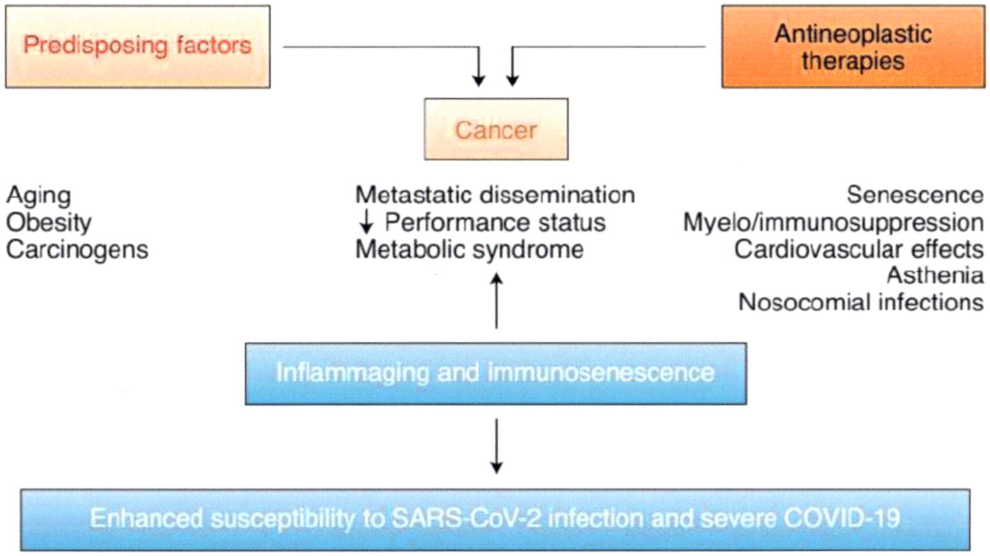

Fig. (10). Relationships between cancer and COVID-19 susceptibility.

7. ANTICANCER DRUGS USED TO INCREASE THE VULNERABILITY OF COVID-19

The list of anticancer medicines along with their other details are illustrated in Table **1**.

Table 1. Anticancer drugs used to increase the vulnerability of COVID-19.

Anticancer Therapies	Risk Factor For COVID-19	Side-Effect Mechanism
Bevacizumab	Thrombosis and proteinuria	Increases the permeability of arterial and vascular thrombosis
Mitomycin C	Pulmonary fibrosis and veno-occlusive diseases	Fibroblast
Anti-HER2 agents(trastuzumab)	Congestive heart failure, systolic function	Loss of myocytes
Pembrolizumab	Pneumonitis	Autoimmune destruction
Ipilimumab	Hypophysitis, hepatitis, exacerbation	Immune activation
Sirolimus	Hyperlipidemia, hypophosphatemia	Reduces the secretion of glucose simulated insulin and increases apoptosis
Cabozantinib	Hypertension, heart failure	Mitochondrial dysfunction, cardiac contractile dysfunction

8. PRO-COVID-19 EFFECTS ON CANCER THERAPY

There are several agents utilised to inhibit the growth of COVID-19 infections. Various types of antiviral drugs with antineoplastic properties and anticancer agents are utilised against COVID-19 [65, 66].

8.1. Interferon Therapy

For anticancer therapy, recombinant of IFNγ and INFα2b is are utilised. They are also used in combination with other drugs. The antiviral response of type 1 interferon might be compromised by the coronavirus. These drugs are used in the form of vapour inhalations. Ribavirin, remdesivir and hydroxychloroquine are used for the treatment of COVID-19. The aerosol of IFNγ has demonstrated effectiveness againsttuberculosis. The pulmonary function is done for patients' idiopathic pulmonary fibrosis. The treatment is used against COPD and tuberculosis. The blood in lung cancer patients indicates heavy viral loads. Not only that, cytotoxic therapies are also used for the treatment of COVID-19 (Fig. **11**) [67, 68].

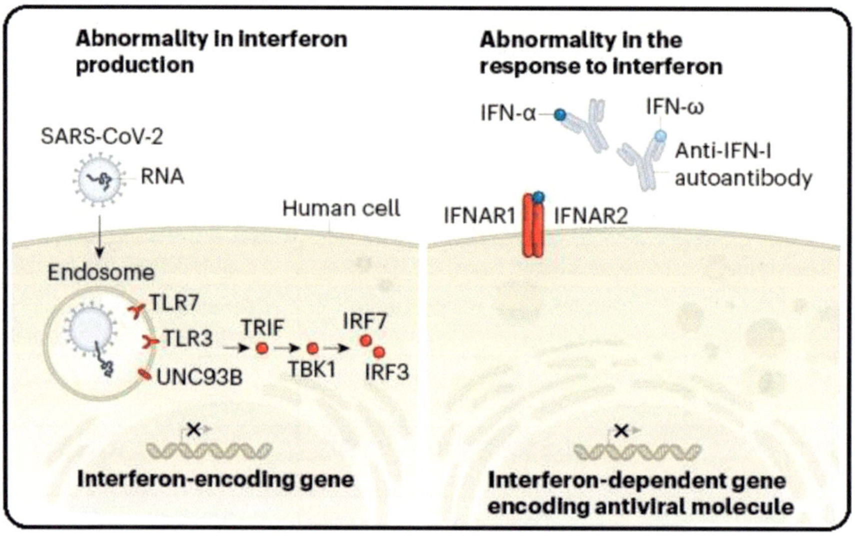

Fig. (11). Interferon Therapy.

8.2. Immune Blockers

The cytotoxic T cell would boost the immunotherapy due to the blockage of immune checkpoints. It is used against neoplastic cells and virus. T cells play the most important role in COVID-19 treatment. In this treatment, the therapeutic exacerbation of disease occurs through T cells that depict lung immunopathology. CTL exhaustion is used for pneumonitis which would eliminate the inflammation of myeloid cells. HLH (hemophagocytic lymphohistiocytosis) displays secondary hemophagocytic response induced by the virus which would prolong macrophages activation (Fig. **12**) [69, 70].

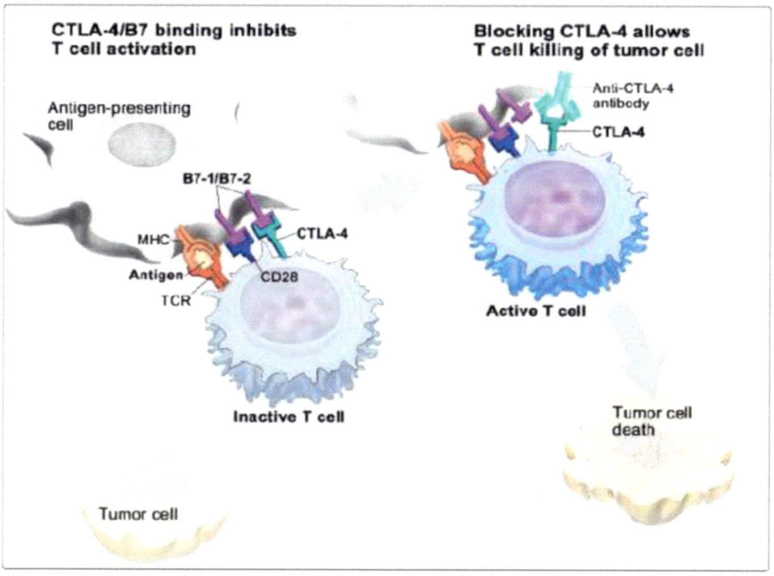

Fig. (12). Immune Blocker.

8.3. JAK– IL-6–STAT3 Blockade

The cytokine release syndrome can cascade the inflammatory action. The monoclonal antibody IL-6R (tocilizumab) is used for the treatment of COVID-19 because it has greater effect on the improvement of clinical and radiological activity. It also helps to restore the T cell that is associated with adaptive immunity. Furthermore, rheumatoid arthritis would reduce the neutrophile count for chronic patients. Neutrophiles would inflame the lungs which leads to haematopoiesis, worsening the symptoms of COVID-19. In overt pneumonia, IL-6R might block the trail assessment (Fig. **13**) [71, 72].

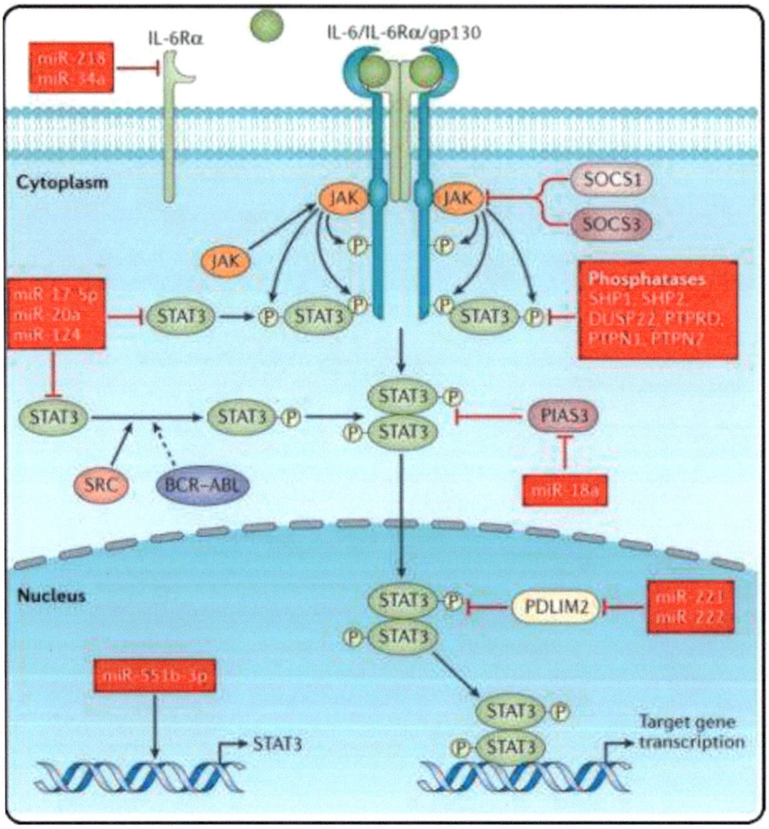

Fig. (13). JAK-IL6-STAT3 Blockade.

8.4. Androgen-Deprivation Therapy

TMPRSS2 expression would be enhanced by signalling the androgen-receptor. It increases the vulnerability, mainly among males who are affected by COVID-19. TMPRSS2 could be reduced by ADT(androgen-deprivation therapy). T would protect the viral entry due to the combination of drugs. COVID-19 prophylactic therapy would be able to evaluate the medications through the combination of ADT with LH-RH modulators (Fig. **14**) [73, 74].

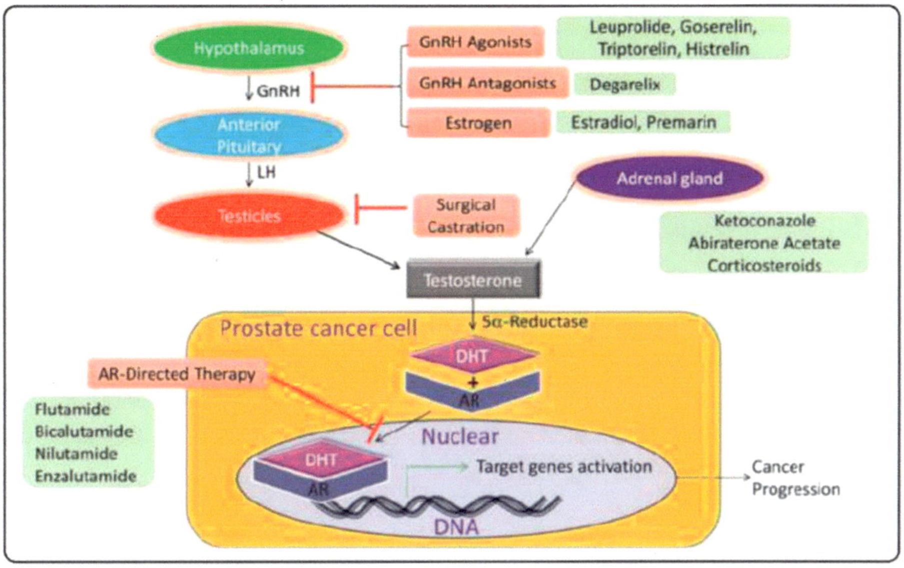

Fig. (14). Androgen-Deprivation Therapy.

8.5. Other Small Molecules

HCQ (hydroxychloroquine) is utilised for the treatment of autophagy-dependent cancer. It is able to reduce the infection of the virus and the effects of the drugs. It is also used in the treatment of cancer. There are other drugs with small molecules and possess anti-cancer and anti-COVID-19 activity. They can inhibit the infection by elongating the factor 1A and initiating the eukaryotic factor 4A [75, 76].

8.6. ANTIVIRAL DRUGS THAT HAVE SHOWN ANTITUMOR EFFECT AGAINST COVID-19

The details of antiviral drugs are illustrated in Table **2**.

Table 2. Antiviral drugs that have shown antitumor effect against covid-19.

Antiviral Drugs	Anti-CoV-2 Effect	Anticancer Mechanism
Ritonavir	No effecthad taken place	inhibit chymotrypsin, suppress BCL-2 andNF-kβ
Lopinavir	Produces effects at a high dose	Inhibit proliferation and induct cell signalling
Nafamostat	Produces effects	Apoptosis may be dependent on induced mitochondria
Penciclovir	Produces effects	S phase cells can be accumulated and death of apoptotic

(Table 2) cont.....

Antiviral drugs	Anti-CoV-2 Effect	Anticancer Mechanism
Ribavirin	Produces effects at a high dose	Cervical cancer cells may be depleted, cell death, inhibition of growth, immunotherapy effects

9. RISK FACTORS OF CARDIOVASCULAR SYSTEM AND COVID-19

9.1. Cardiovascular Comorbidities Underlying

Comorbidity of cardiovascular system can affect COVID-19 patients. In China, CVD is recognised as the most important risk factor. Hypertension and diabetes are said to be the highest comorbidities than any other diseases. Based on the study, 72% to 80% of patients were admitted in ICU. Other studies also have shown that about 48% to 50% COVID-19 patients have comorbidities of hypertension and diabetes [77, 78].

9.2. Cardiovascular Manifestations of Diverse

Pneumonia is the main manifestation of COVID-19 which can lead to myocardial injury, thromboembolism and arrhythmias. Some of the first clinical manifestations of COVID-19 which have high mortality are cardiac syndrome and fever.

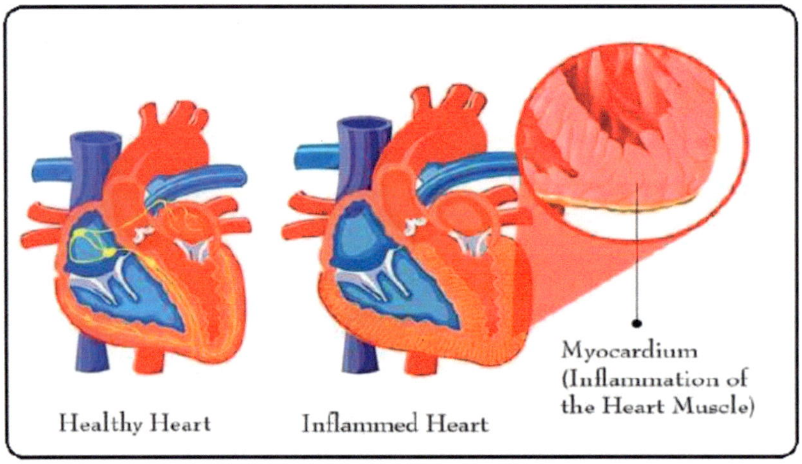

Fig. (15). myocarditis.

9.2.1. Myocarditis

Biomarker and ECG (electrocardiogram) are used to elevate patients' acute myocardial injury. The worst prognosis is often associated with the presence of myocardial injury. Some reports have shown that 5 to 10 patients have myocardial injury with high level of cardiac troponin I. In cardiac injury, 5-fold is increased by mechanical ventilation while mortality is increased by 11-fold.. 37% to 38% death rate of COVID-19 have an elevated level of cardiac troponin T (Fig. **15**). The myocardial injury marker would predicate the risk factor in-hospital mortality [81, 82].

9.2.2. Cardiovascular Diseases and Covid-19 Bidirectional Interaction

High mortality of COVID-19 comes with cardiovascular comorbidity. There are drugs that can be used to reduce the cardiovascular risk and susceptibility in COVID-19. COVID-19 has viral pneumonia which can induce the cardiovascular manifestations. Furthermore, the myocardial injury in COVID-19 shows high risk of mortality. Hydroxychloroquine and azithromycin are used for the pro-arrhythmic effects (Fig. **16**) [83, 84].

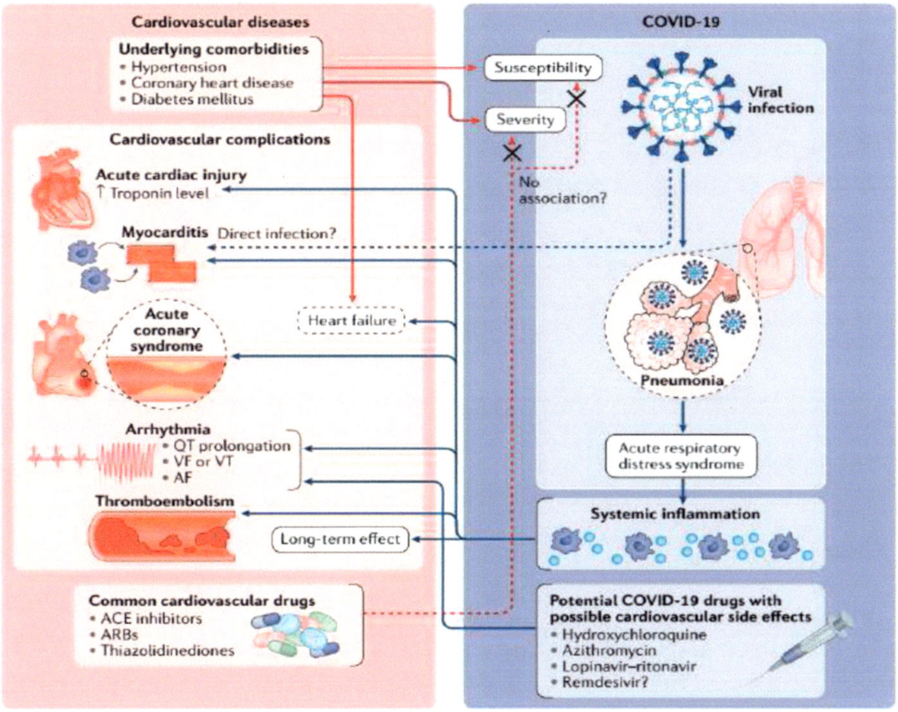

Fig. (16). Bidirectional interaction between COVID-19 and cardiovascular diseases.

9.2.3. Acute Coronary Syndrome

There are several countries with active cases of COVID-19 that are dealing with ACS that is triggered by the virus which induces chest pain. Percutaneous intervention coronary diseases with elevated ST segments have increased among COVID-19 patients in New York and Italy. Coronary angiography depicts culprit lesion with revascularization. The elevation of ST segment in myocardial infarction is the first clinical manifestation of COVID-19 (Fig. **17**) [85, 86].

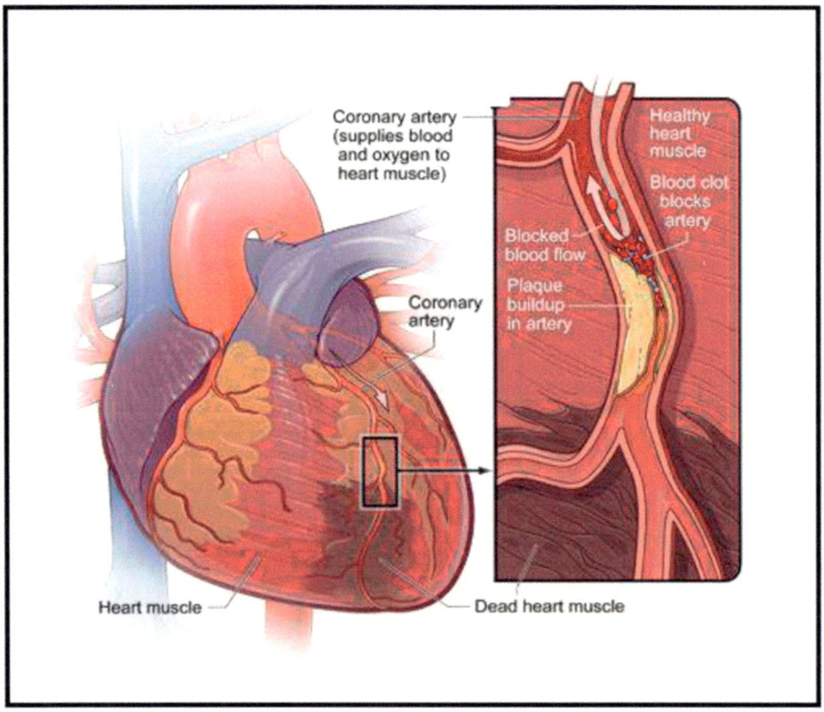

Fig. (17). Acute Coronary Syndrome.

9.2.4. Heart Failure

Heart failure is one of the complications of COVID-19. Patients identified with amino-terminal pro-B-type natriuretic peptide have increased. COVID-19 patients with pre-existing comorbidities will have higher risk of heart failure. Heart failure can occur when the diastolic function is reduced. It can trigger high fever, renal function impaired and excessive hydration. For the detection of COVID-19 among patients with heart failure, the ejection fraction and cardiac MRI are utilised. COVID-19 also can trigger acute myocardial injury and ACS. The stress induced cardiomyopathy can be triggered during the early stage of COVID-19. The cytokine related myocardial dysfunction will also occur in cardiac dysfunction. Respiratory and pneumonia also can occur in the bilateral and lower lung distribution (Fig. **18**) [87 - 89].

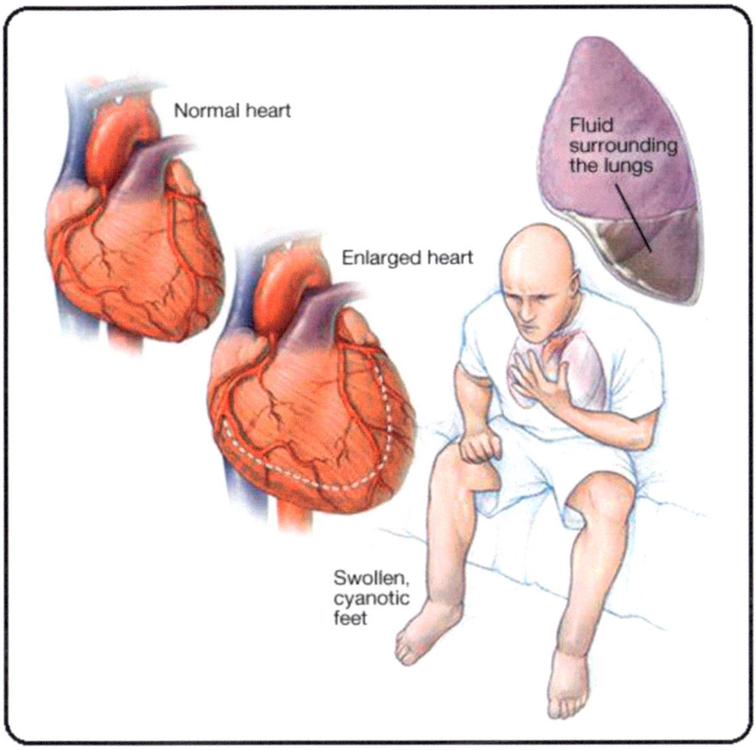

Fig. (18). Heart Failure.

9.2.5. Cardiac Arrest

Cardiac arrest is a common manifestation of COVID-19. The palpitations of the heart are the main symptoms of COVID-19. 17% to 20% of cardiac arrhythmia have been reported in Wuhan, China. Due to this, ventricular tachycardia and fibrillation are developed to elevate the level of troponin T. Nonetheless, sudden cardiac arrest cases have been reported at in-hospital and out-hospital, all over the world (Fig. **19**).

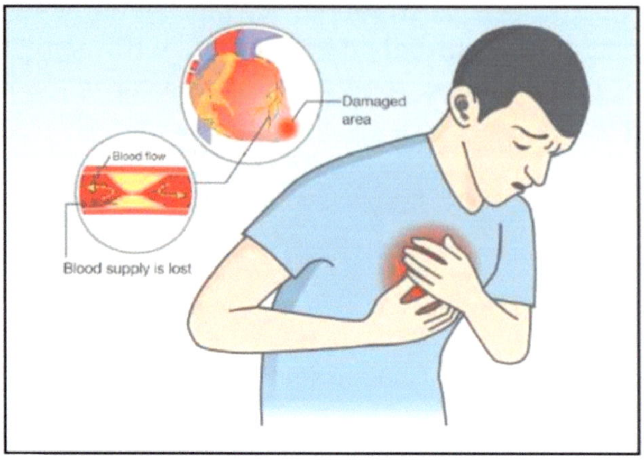

Fig (19). Cardiac Arrest.

9.2.6. Coagulation and Thrombosis

Thromboembolic is associated with the coagulation abnormalities of COVID-19. As such, the d-dimer would reduce the platelet counts and prolong the time of prothrombin therefore, patients with D-dimer could elevate the infection. Due to this, the death rate has increased by 18-fold. Apart from that, patients' level of fibrinogen and factor VIII have increased, further suggesting intravascular coagulation abnormalities. Furthermore, it also can develop the cardiovascular manifestation of COVID-19. Among critically ill patients, venous thromboembolism has induced deep vein pulmonary embolism. This particular scenario has been observed in New York and Italy in which these large vessels have depicted ischaemic stroke and acute limb ischaemia (Fig. **20**) [92, 93].

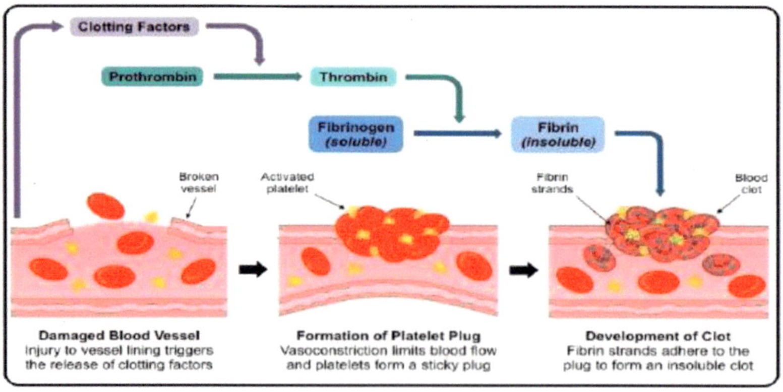

Fig. (20). Coagulation and Thrombosis.

9.2.7. Kawasaki Disease

Children are less susceptible to COVID-19 and majority would only contracted mild symptoms when infected. The virus however can cause severe inflammation among paediatric patients. Of late, Kawasaki disease among eight-year old children has been reported in several countries. The symptoms of this disease include fever, rashes, oedema and GIT syndromes. It also can form hyper inflammatory syndrome (Fig. **21**) [94, 95]. It is important to note that the occurrence of Kawasaki disease among children can increase by 30-fold.

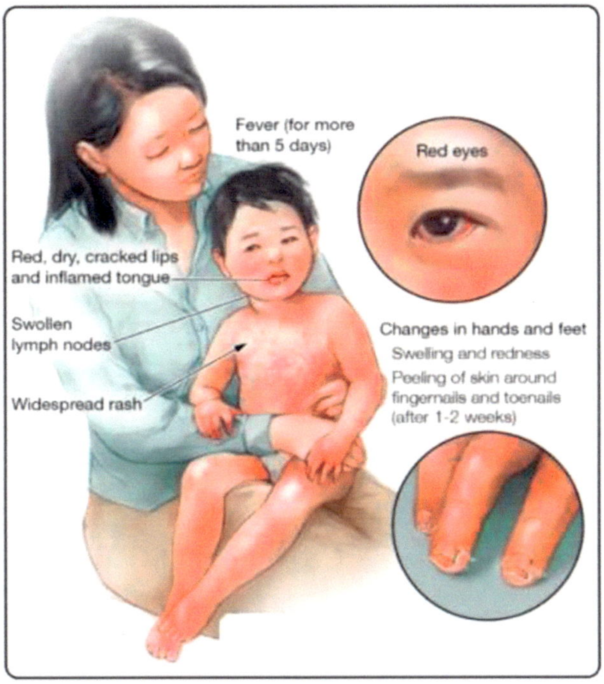

Fig. (21). Kawasaki Disease.

9.2.8. Immunocompromised Patients

Patients with low immunity have higher risk of contracting COVID-19 which is evident among cancer patients and those with weak cardiovascular system. Patients who have undergone heart transplantation also have higher risk of contracting the virus. Certain countries that have a great number of organ transplantations like USA and China have higher risk of being infected with COVID-19. Immunosuppression would preserve the allograft function thus, the treatment might cause harmful effects on the progression of diseases (Fig. **22**) [96, 97].

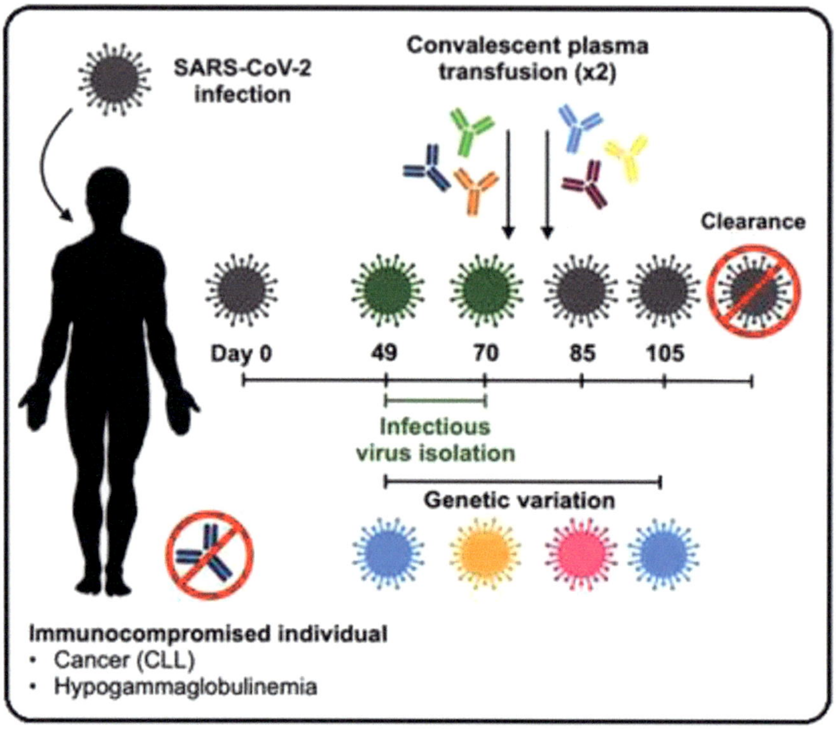

Fig. (22). Immunocompromised Patients.

10. ACE2 MANIFESTATIONS IN CARDIOVASCULAR DISEASES

COVID-19 can cause cardiovascular injury. ACE2 is an important factor in the biological mechanism of tissues specific infection. The S protein would bind with the ACE2 human proteins. Then, these proteins would bind with the viral S protein. RAAS contains ACE2 and it is used in the development of diabetes, hypertension and heart failure. ACE2 is highly expressed in lungs and kidney. The data sequencing of RNA is expressed in the heart and coronary arteries. The cardiomyocytes of single cell RNA sequencing data have revealed that the expression would lower the pericytes and nor- cardiomyocytes in TMPRSS2. Therefore, the virus would enter through the endocytic pathway with the high expression of cathepsin B and L and directly affect the cardiovascular cells (Fig. **23**) [98, 99].

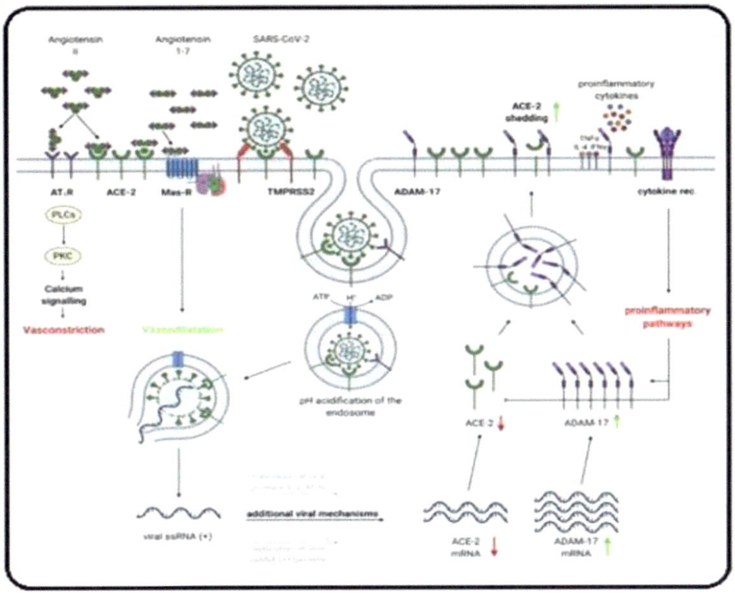

Fig. (23). ACE2 Manifestations in Cardiovascular Diseases.

10.1. ACE2 DOWNREGULATION FOR COVID 19

COVID-19 cell is expressed into the downregulation of ACE2. Once the infection reaches the heart, the level of ACE2 is reduced. The cardiac contractility will reduce the knockout of ACE2. The gene is encoded and upregulated into the molecule and cytokines like IL-6 and CCL2. ACE2 depicts protective effects in the lungs. ACE2 is expressed by the alveolar epithelial type II cells. The cells also produce the surfactant proteins and reduce the surface tension. Furthermore, they also prevent the alveoli from collapsing. The recombinant ACE2 is used in the treatment of lung diseases which would result in the downregulation of ACE2, therefore, leading to cardiac dysfunction and atherosclerosis (Fig. **24**) [100, 101].

10.2. THERAPEUTIC TARGET ACE2

RAAS consists of angiotensin II effector molecule which can be regulated in other types of diseases. This is beneficial for the target treatment in cardiovascular disorders. Angiotensin-II is converted into angiotensin which can inactivate ACE2. S proteins bind directly to ACE2 and have a higher affinity to COVID-19. These recombinant ACE2s would prevent the infection by forming a decoy. rhACE2 clinical grade is utilised to reduce the infection of COVID-19 and protect the CVDs (Fig. **25**) [102, 103].

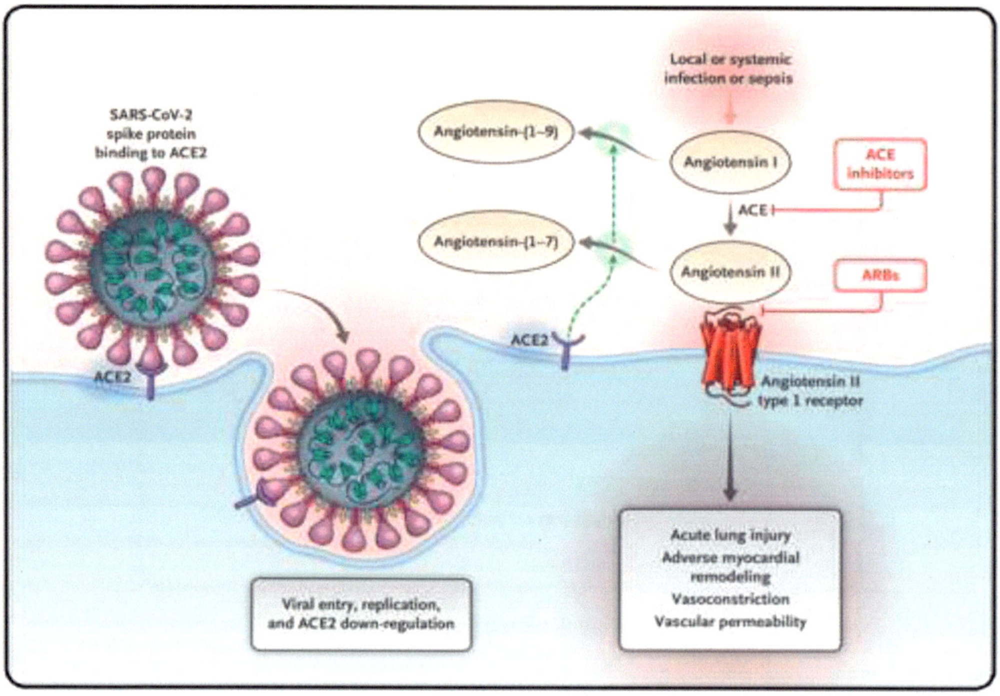

Fig. (24). ACE2 downregulation for covid 19.

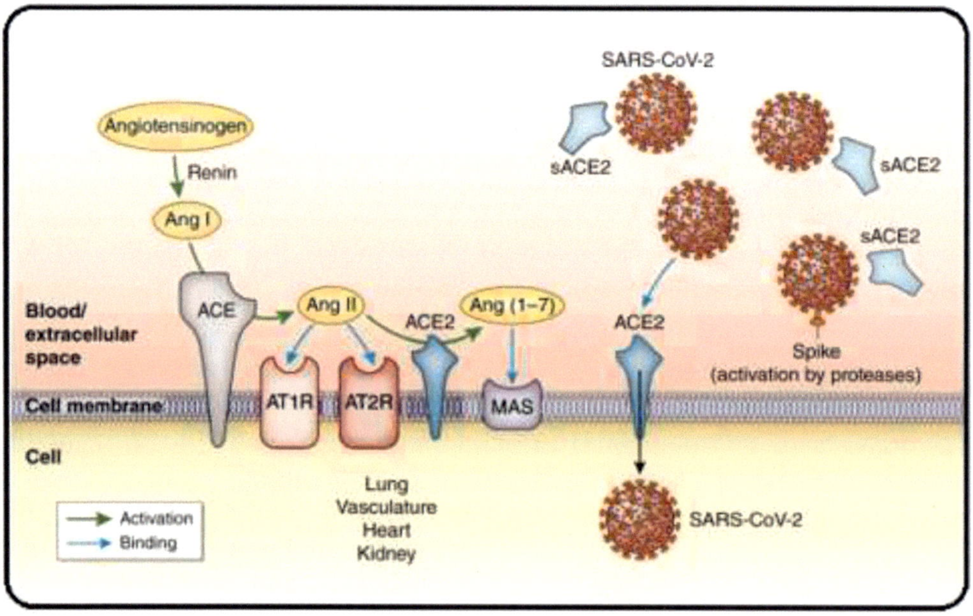

Fig. (25). COVID-19 Infection Targeted ACE2.

10.3. COVID 19 BROAD TISSUE TROPISM

COVID-19 can infect lungs and respiratory tract. It can manifest extra pulmonary complications like liver damage and renal dysfunction. The viral pneumonia would induce hyperinflammation. RNA has been detected by reverse transcription PCR at a high concentration. COVID-19 also may have mechanistically broad tissue tropism which depicts the instability of S proteins (Fig. **26**) [104, 105].

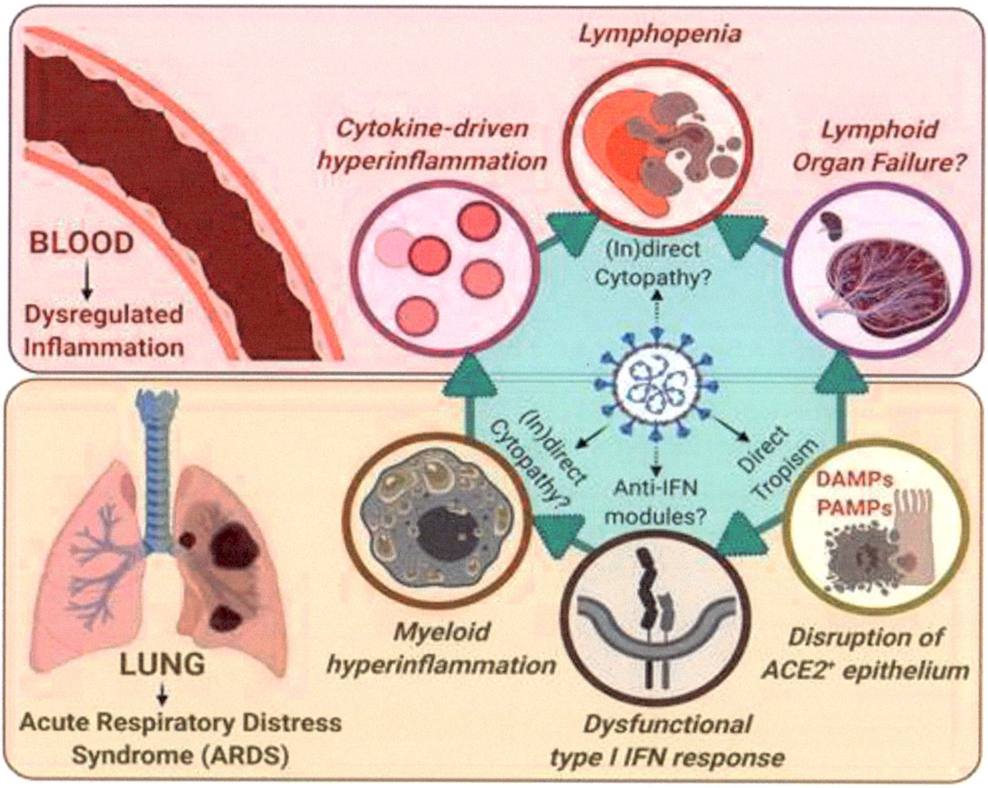

Fig. (26). COVID 19 Broad Tissue Tropism.

10.4. ENDOTHELIAL CELLS FOR VIRAL TARGETING

COVID-19 virus directly targets the endothelial cells. Due to this, patients who had succumbed to the virus had multi-organ failures. Cells inflammation would cause endotheliitis and depict the apoptotic bodies in high concentration. The small intestine may be a prominent endotheliitis of submucosal vessels in large apoptotic bodies. It can infect the endothethial cells, thus, leading to inflammation in the endothelium (Fig. **27**) [106, 107].

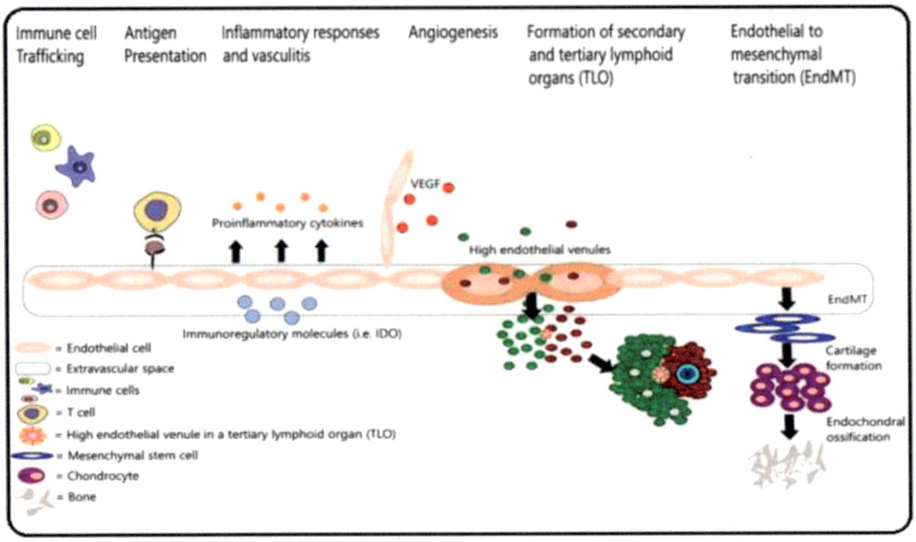

Fig. (27). Endothelial Cells for Viral Targeting.

10.5. DRUG–DISEASE INTERACTIONS

For the prevention of COVID-19, ACE inhibitors and angiotensin II receptor blocker are utilised (Fig. **28**) [108, 109].

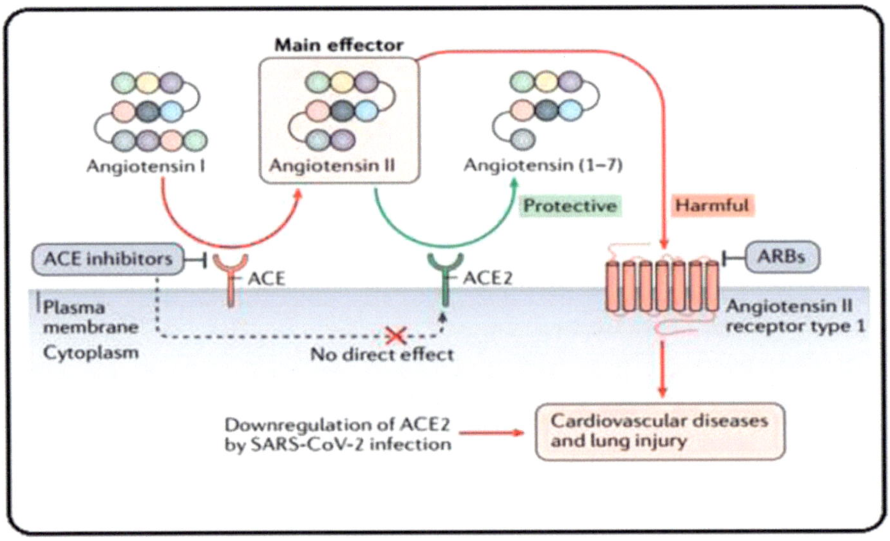

Fig (28). Drug-Disease Interaction.

10.5.1. RAAS Inhibitors On Covid 19

COVID-19 affects ACE2 receptors by upregulating the cell surface. Due to this, ARBs can be inhibited by increasing the ACE2 expression. This method is utilised for the treatment of CVD and hypertensions. Due to the effect of COVID-19, RAAS antagonist is recommended to be utilised as it is not associated with positive COVID-19. RAAS would inhibit the ACE2 controversial and target ACE and ACE2 inhibitors. Moreover, angiotensin I is converted into angiotensin II by ACE while angiotensin II is degraded into angiotensin by ACE2. Therefore, RAAS is believed to have indirect effects on ACE inhibitors (Fig. **29**) [110, 111].

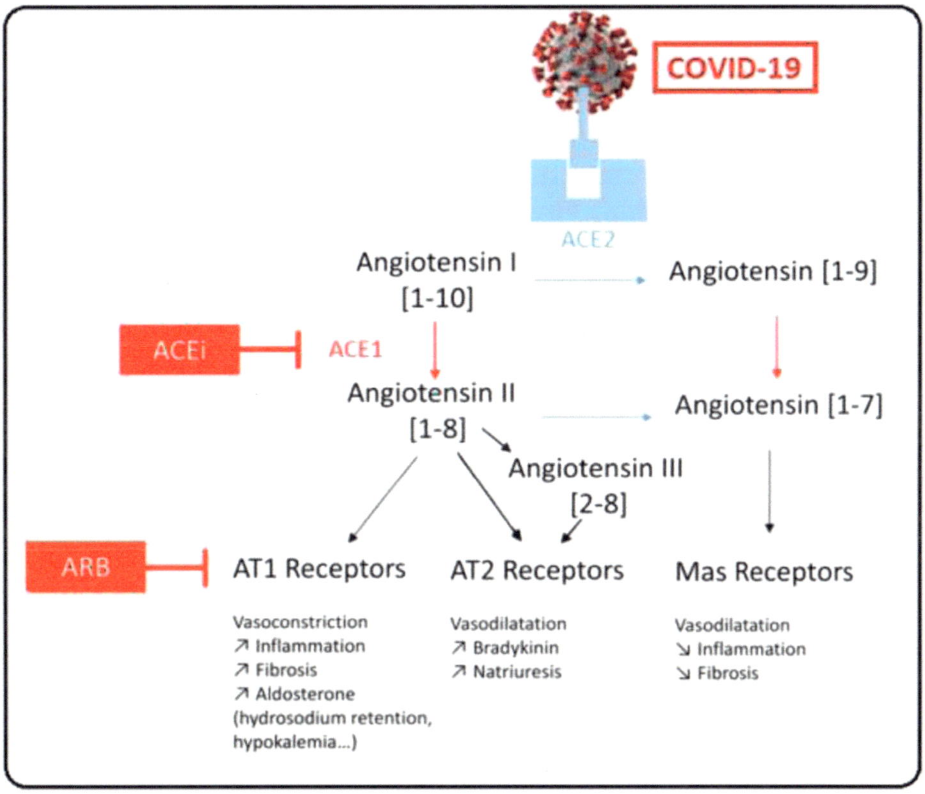

Fig. (29). RAAS inhibitors on covid 19.

10.5.2. Antiviral Drugs for Cardiovascular Effects

Several types of drugs are currently utilised for the prevention and treatment of COVID-19. However, the development of effective drugs has consumed a lot of time [112].

10.5.3. Hydroxychloroquine and Azithromycin

Chloroquine and hydroxychloroquine are used for the treatment of COVID-19 to block the virus from entering through the endosomal pathway. They would inhibit the glycosylation in the host cells. They also demonstrate proteolytic and endolytic acidification. The production of cytokine is attenuated and mediated by the immune system. It inhibits the lysosomal and autophagy activity. Furthermore, hydroxychloroquine would help in the clearance of coronavirus in the cells. The combination of Azithromycin and HCQ has shown better virus clearance [113, 114].

10.5.4. Remdesivir

Remdesivir is used for the treatment of COVID-19 as it has a broad-spectrum antiviral activity to target the RdRP. Previously, this particular drug is mainly used for the treatment of Ebola virus. It helps to lower the virus load in pulmonary function. China in particular has been utilising the drug and has had better results than other drugs. Not only that, it also provides faster recovery period [115, 116].

10.5.5. Lopinavir–ritonavir

These drugs are mainly used for the treatment of HIV infections to inhibit the protease activity. Lopinavir helps to inhibit cytochrome P450. Continuous usage of the drugs can lead to GIT disturbance. These combinations would also interact with CV drugs and metabolised cytochrome P450. They are also used for antiplatelet drugs and anticoagulants [117, 118].

CONCLUSION

The current situation of COVID-19 has affected the health of millions people around the world. The virus also has mainly affected unhealthy and unfit people as well as patients with cardiovascular and cancer diseases. Patients with cancer and CVDs have higher risk due to factors such as age, obesity, smoking habit and other comorbidities. The antineoplastic therapy would help to debilitate the immune system which would cause immune-senescence and inflammation. The risk factor of COVID-19 is elucidated. The morbidity and mortality of COVID-19 patients with cancer and CVD may be affected with viral diseases [119, 120]. Not only that, it also may affect the treatment of both diseases. A strong therapeutic strategy is currently utilised to improve the diseases condition. Certain types of drugs are effective to inhibit the effect of COVID-19.Dual therapy also is used against COVID-19 infection. There are several benefits of IL6R. Neutralisation of COVID-19 antibodies is a passive transfer which can moderate the stage of COVID-19. Severe COVID-19 would be able to protect the antiviral T cells and have an active vaccination. Vaccines that have been developed however should undergo large scale of clinical trials to improve their effectiveness and safety [121, 122].

The pandemic has significantly altered everyone's life. Due to this, many tests have been conducted to improve the health care system. Some precautions have been implemented such as social distancing, lockdown and reducing physical activity to prevent widespread of infections [123, 124].

CONSENT FOR PUBLICATION

Not applicable.

CONFLICT OF INTEREST

The author declares no conflict of interest, financial or otherwise.

ACKNOWLEDGEMENTS

Declared none.

REFERENCES

[1] Zhou P, Yang XL, Wang XG, *et al.* A pneumonia outbreak associated with a new coronavirus of probable bat origin. Nature 2020; 579(7798): 270-3.
[http://dx.doi.org/10.1038/s41586-020-2012-7] [PMID: 32015507]

[2] Wu F, Zhao S, Yu B, *et al.* A new coronavirus associated with human respiratory disease in China. Nature 2020; 579(7798): 265-9.
[http://dx.doi.org/10.1038/s41586-020-2008-3] [PMID: 32015508]

[3] Lu R, Zhao X, Li J, *et al.* Genomic characterisation and epidemiology of 2019 novel coronavirus: implications for virus origins and receptor binding. Lancet 2020; 395(10224): 565-74.
[http://dx.doi.org/10.1016/S0140-6736(20)30251-8] [PMID: 32007145]

[4] Hoffmann M, Kleine-Weber H, Schroeder S, *et al.* SARS-CoV-2 cell entry depends on ACE2 and TMPRSS2 and is blocked by a clinically proven protease inhibitor. Cell 2020; 181(2): 271-280.e8.
[http://dx.doi.org/10.1016/j.cell.2020.02.052] [PMID: 32142651]

[5] Tay MZ, Poh CM, Rénia L, MacAry PA, Ng LFP. The trinity of COVID-19: immunity, inflammation and intervention. Nat Rev Immunol 2020; 20(6): 363-74.
[http://dx.doi.org/10.1038/s41577-020-0311-8] [PMID: 32346093]

[6] Bikdeli B, Madhavan MV, Jimenez D, *et al.* COVID-19 and thrombotic or thromboembolic disease: implications for prevention, antithrombotic therapy, and follow-up: JACC stateof-the-art review. J Am Coll Cardiol 2020; 75(23): 2950-73.
[http://dx.doi.org/10.1016/j.jacc.2020.04.031] [PMID: 32311448]

[7] Connors JM, Levy JH. Thromboinflammation and the hypercoagulability of COVID-19. J Thromb

Haemost 2020; 18(7): 1559-61.
[http://dx.doi.org/10.1111/jth.14849] [PMID: 32302453]

[8] Andersen KG, Rambaut A, Lipkin WI, Holmes EC, Garry RF. The proximal origin of SARS-CoV-2. Nat Med 2020; 26(4): 450-2.
[http://dx.doi.org/10.1038/s41591-020-0820-9] [PMID: 32284615]

[9] Wrapp D, Wang N, Corbett KS, *et al.* Cryo-EM structure of the 2019-nCoV spike in the prefusion conformation. Science 2020; 367(6483): 1260-3.
[http://dx.doi.org/10.1126/science.abb2507] [PMID: 32075877]

[10] Walls AC, Park YJ, Tortorici MA, Wall A, McGuire AT, Veesler D. Structure, function, and antigenicity of the SARS-CoV-2 spike glycoprotein. Cell 2020; 181(2): 281-292.e6.
[http://dx.doi.org/10.1016/j.cell.2020.02.058] [PMID: 32155444]

[11] Wan Y, Shang J, Graham R, Baric RS, Li F. Receptor recognition by the novel coronavirus from Wuhan: an analysis based on decade-long structural studies of SARS coronavirus. J Virol 2020; 94(7): e00127-20.
[http://dx.doi.org/10.1128/JVI.00127-20] [PMID: 31996437]

[12] Madjid M, Safavi-Naeini P, Solomon SD, Vardeny O. Potential effects of coronaviruses on the cardiovascular system: a review. JAMA Cardiol 2020; 5(7): 831-40.
[http://dx.doi.org/10.1001/jamacardio.2020.1286] [PMID: 32219363]

[13] Clerkin KJ, Fried JA, Raikhelkar J, *et al.* COVID-19 and cardiovascular disease. Circulation 2020; 141(20): 1648-55.
[http://dx.doi.org/10.1161/CIRCULATIONAHA.120.046941] [PMID: 32200663]

[14] Driggin E, Madhavan MV, Bikdeli B, *et al.* Cardiovascular considerations for patients, health care workers, and health systems during the COVID-19 pandemic. J Am Coll Cardiol 2020; 75(18): 2352-71.
[http://dx.doi.org/10.1016/j.jacc.2020.03.031] [PMID: 32201335]

[15] Zheng YY, Ma YT, Zhang JY, Xie X. COVID-19 and the cardiovascular system. Nat Rev Cardiol 2020; 17(5): 259-60.
[http://dx.doi.org/10.1038/s41569-020-0360-5] [PMID: 32139904]

[16] Han Y, Zeng H, Jiang H, *et al.* CSC expert consensus on principles of clinical management of patients with severe emergent cardiovascular diseases during the COVID-19 epidemic. Circulation 2020; 141(20): e810-6.
[http://dx.doi.org/10.1161/CIRCULATIONAHA.120.047011] [PMID: 32216640]

[17] Huang C, Wang Y, Li X, *et al.* Clinical features of patients infected with 2019 novel coronavirus in Wuhan, China. Lancet 2020; 395(10223): 497-506.
[http://dx.doi.org/10.1016/S0140-6736(20)30183-5] [PMID: 31986264]

[18] Wang D, Hu B, Hu C, *et al.* Clinical characteristics of 138 hospitalized patients with 2019 novel coronavirus infected pneumonia in Wuhan, China. JAMA 2021; 325(11): 1113.
[PMID: 32031570]

[19] Zhou F, Yu T, Du R, *et al.* Clinical course and risk factors for mortality of adult inpatients with COVID-19 in Wuhan, China: a retrospective cohort study. Lancet 2020; 395(10229): 1054-62.
[http://dx.doi.org/10.1016/S0140-6736(20)30566-3] [PMID: 32171076]

[20] Guan W, Ni Z, Hu Y, *et al.* Clinical characteristics of coronavirus disease 2019 in China. N Engl J Med 2020; 382(18): 1708-20.
[http://dx.doi.org/10.1056/NEJMoa2002032] [PMID: 32109013]

[21] Wu Z, McGoogan JM. Characteristics of and important lessons from the coronavirus disease 2019 (COVID-19) outbreak in China. JAMA 2020; 323(13): 1239-42.
[http://dx.doi.org/10.1001/jama.2020.2648] [PMID: 32091533]

[22] Ruan Q, Yang K, Wang W, Jiang L, Song J. Clinical predictors of mortality due to COVID-19 based

on an analysis of data of 150 patients from Wuhan, China. Intensive Care Med 2020; 46(5): 846-8. [http://dx.doi.org/10.1007/s00134-020-05991-x] [PMID: 32125452]

[23] Shi S, Qin M, Shen B, *et al.* Association of cardiac injury with mortality in hospitalized patients with COVID-19 in Wuhan, China. JAMA Cardiol 2020; 5(7): 802-10. [http://dx.doi.org/10.1001/jamacardio.2020.0950] [PMID: 32211816]

[24] Guo T, Fan Y, Chen M, *et al.* Cardiovascular implications of fatal outcomes of patients with coronavirus disease 2019 (COVID-19). JAMA Cardiol 2020; 5(7): 811-8. [http://dx.doi.org/10.1001/jamacardio.2020.1017] [PMID: 32219356]

[25] Shi S, Qin M, Cai Y, *et al.* Characteristics and clinical significance of myocardial injury in patients with severe coronavirus disease 2019. Eur Heart J 2020; 41(22): 2070-9. [http://dx.doi.org/10.1093/eurheartj/ehaa408] [PMID: 32391877]

[26] Riphagen S, Gomez X, Gonzalez-Martinez C, Wilkinson N, Theocharis P. Hyperinflammatory shock in children during COVID-19 pandemic. Lancet 2020; 395(10237): 1607-8. [http://dx.doi.org/10.1016/S0140-6736(20)31094-1] [PMID: 32386565]

[27] Yin W, Mao C, Luan X, *et al.* Structural basis for inhibition of the RNA-dependent RNA polymerase from SARS-CoV-2 by remdesivir. Science 2020; 368(6498): 1499-504. [http://dx.doi.org/10.1126/science.abc1560] [PMID: 32358203]

[28] Dai W, Zhang B, Jiang XM, *et al.* Structure-based design of antiviral drug candidates targeting the SARS-CoV-2 main protease. Science 2020; 368(6497): 1331-5. [http://dx.doi.org/10.1126/science.abb4489] [PMID: 32321856]

[29] Cui J, Li F, Shi ZL. Origin and evolution of pathogenic coronaviruses. Nat Rev Microbiol 2019; 17(3): 181-92. [http://dx.doi.org/10.1038/s41579-018-0118-9] [PMID: 30531947]

[30] Du L, He Y, Zhou Y, Liu S, Zheng BJ, Jiang S. The spike protein of SARS-CoV — a target for vaccine and therapeutic development. Nat Rev Microbiol 2009; 7(3): 226-36. [http://dx.doi.org/10.1038/nrmicro2090] [PMID: 19198616]

[31] Ge XY, Li JL, Yang XL, *et al.* Isolation and characterization of a bat SARS-like coronavirus that uses the ACE2 receptor. Nature 2013; 503(7477): 535-8. [http://dx.doi.org/10.1038/nature12711] [PMID: 24172901]

[32] On YMB, Flamholz A, Phillips R, Milo R. SARS-CoV-2 (COVID-19) by the numbers. 2020; 9: e57309.

[33] Masson P, Hulo C, De Castro E, *et al.* ViralZone: recent updates to the virus knowledge resource. Nucleic Acids Res 2013; 41(Database issue): D579-83. [PMID: 23193299]

[34] Lurie N, Saville M, Hatchett R, Halton J. Developing COVID-19 vaccines at pandemic speed. N Engl J Med 2020; 382(21): 1969-73. [http://dx.doi.org/10.1056/NEJMp2005630] [PMID: 32227757]

[35] Callaway E. The race for coronavirus vaccines: a graphical guide. Nature 2020; 580(7805): 576-7. [http://dx.doi.org/10.1038/d41586-020-01221-y] [PMID: 32346146]

[36] Suthar MS, Zimmerman MG, Kauffman RC, *et al.* Rapid generation of neutralizing antibody responses in COVID-19 patients. Cell Rep Med 2020; 1(3): 100040. [http://dx.doi.org/10.1016/j.xcrm.2020.100040] [PMID: 32835303]

[37] Wang c, Li W, Drabek D, *et al.* A human monoclonal antibody blocking SARS-CoV-2 infection. Nat. Commun. 2020; 11: 225.

[38] Ho T, Wu S, Chen J, Li C, Hsiang C. Emodin blocks the SARS coronavirus spike protein and angiotensin-converting enzyme 2 interaction. Antiviral Res 2007; 74(2): 92-101. [http://dx.doi.org/10.1016/j.antiviral.2006.04.014] [PMID: 16730806]

[39] Robson B. COVID-19 Coronavirus spike protein analysis for synthetic vaccines, a peptidomimetic antagonist, and therapeutic drugs, and analysis of a proposed achilles' heel conserved region to minimize probability of escape mutations and drug resistance. Comput Biol Med 2020; 121: 103749-9. [http://dx.doi.org/10.1016/j.compbiomed.2020.103749] [PMID: 32568687]

[40] Green KY, Chanock RM, Kapikan AZ. Human caliciviruses. In: Knipe DM, Howley PM, Eds. Fields virology 4th ed. 2001; 841-74.

[41] Sanders JM, Monogue ML, Jodlowski TZ, Cutrell JB. Pharmacologic treatments for coronavirus disease 2019 (COVID-19): a review. JAMA 2020; 323(18): 1824-36. [http://dx.doi.org/10.1001/jama.2020.6019] [PMID: 32282022]

[42] Li G, De Clercq E. Therapeutic options for the 2019 novel coronavirus (2019-nCoV). Nat Rev Drug Discov 2020; 19(3): 149-50. [http://dx.doi.org/10.1038/d41573-020-00016-0] [PMID: 32127666]

[43] Li SS, Cheng C, Fu C, *et al.* Left ventricular performance in patients with severe acute respiratory syndrome: a 30-day echocardiographic follow-up study. Circulation 2003; 108(15): 1798-803. [http://dx.doi.org/10.1161/01.CIR.0000094737.21775.32] [PMID: 14504188]

[44] Peiris JSM, Chu CM, Cheng VCC, *et al.* Clinical progression and viral load in a community outbreak of coronavirus-associated SARS pneumonia: a prospective study. Lancet 2003; 361(9371): 1767-72. [http://dx.doi.org/10.1016/S0140-6736(03)13412-5] [PMID: 12781535]

[45] CDC Weekly C. Vital surveillances: the epidemiological characteristics of an outbreak of 2019 novel coronavirus diseases (COVID-19) — China, 2020. China CDC Weekly 2020; 2(8): 113-22. [http://dx.doi.org/10.46234/ccdcw2020.032] [PMID: 34594836]

[46] Grasselli G, Zangrillo A, Zanella A, *et al.* Baseline characteristics and outcomes of 1591 patients infected with SARS-CoV-2 admitted to ICUs of the Lombardy region, Italy. JAMA 2020; 323(16): 1574-81. [http://dx.doi.org/10.1001/jama.2020.5394] [PMID: 32250385]

[47] Goyal P, Choi JJ, Pinheiro LC, *et al.* Clinical characteristics of COVID-19 in New York City. N Engl J Med 2020; 382(24): 2372-4. [http://dx.doi.org/10.1056/NEJMc2010419] [PMID: 32302078]

[48] Arentz M, Yim E, Klaff L, *et al.* Characteristics and outcomes of 21 critically ill patients with COVID-19 in Washington state. JAMA 2020; 323(16): 1612-4. [http://dx.doi.org/10.1001/jama.2020.4326] [PMID: 32191259]

[49] Bhatraju PK, Ghassemieh BJ, Nichols M, *et al.* COVID-19 in critically ill patients in the Seattle region — case series. N Engl J Med 2020; 382(21): 2012-22. [http://dx.doi.org/10.1056/NEJMoa2004500] [PMID: 32227758]

[50] Onder G, Rezza G, Brusaferro S. Case-fatality rate and characteristics of patients dying in relation to COVID-19 in Italy. JAMA 2020; 323(18): 1775-6. [http://dx.doi.org/10.1001/jama.2020.4683] [PMID: 32203977]

[51] Richardson S, Hirsch JS, Narasimhan M, *et al.* Presenting characteristics, comorbidities, and outcomes among 5700 patients hospitalized with COVID-19 in the New York City area. JAMA 2020; 323(20): 2052-9. [http://dx.doi.org/10.1001/jama.2020.6775] [PMID: 32320003]

[52] Stefanini GG, Montorfano M, Trabattoni D, *et al.* ST-elevation myocardial infarction in patients with COVID-19: clinical and angiographic outcomes. Circulation 2020; 141(25): 2113-6. [http://dx.doi.org/10.1161/CIRCULATIONAHA.120.047525] [PMID: 32352306]

[53] Deng Q, Hu B, Zhang Y, *et al.* Suspected myocardial injury in patients with COVID-19: Evidence from front-line clinical observation in Wuhan, China. Int J Cardiol 2020; 311: 116-21. [http://dx.doi.org/10.1016/j.ijcard.2020.03.087] [PMID: 32291207]

[54] Wang D, Li S, Jiang J, *et al.* Chinese society of cardiology expert consensus statement on the diagnosis and treatment of adult fulminant myocarditis. Sci China Life Sci 2019; 62(2): 187-202. [http://dx.doi.org/10.1007/s11427-018-9385-3] [PMID: 30519877]

[55] Inciardi RM, Lupi L, Zaccone G, *et al.* Cardiac involvement in a patient with coronavirus disease 2019 (COVID-19). JAMA Cardiol. 2020; 5(7): 819-24.

[56] Hu H, Ma F, Wei X, Fang Y. Coronavirus fulminant myocarditis treated with glucocorticoid and human immunoglobulin. Eur Heart J 2021; 42(2): 206. [http://dx.doi.org/10.1093/eurheartj/ehaa190] [PMID: 32176300]

[57] Xu Z, Shi L, Wang Y, *et al.* Pathological findings of COVID-19 associated with acute respiratory distress syndrome. Lancet Respir Med 2020; 8(4): 420-2. [http://dx.doi.org/10.1016/S2213-2600(20)30076-X] [PMID: 32085846]

[58] Tavazzi G, Pellegrini C, Maurelli M, *et al.* Myocardial localization of coronavirus in COVID-19 cardiogenic shock. Eur J Heart Fail 2020; 22(5): 911-5. [http://dx.doi.org/10.1002/ejhf.1828] [PMID: 32275347]

[59] Wichmann D, Sperhake JP, Lutgehetmann M, *et al.* Autopsy findings and venous thromboembolism in patients with COVID-19. 2020.

[60] Schaller T, Hirschbühl K, Burkhardt K, *et al.* Postmortem examination of patients with COVID-19. JAMA 2020; 323(24): 2518-20. [http://dx.doi.org/10.1001/jama.2020.8907] [PMID: 32437497]

[61] Jiang F, Yang J, Zhang Y, *et al.* Angiotensin-converting enzyme 2 and angiotensin 1–7: novel therapeutic targets. Nat Rev Cardiol 2014; 11(7): 413-26. [http://dx.doi.org/10.1038/nrcardio.2014.59] [PMID: 24776703]

[62] Oudit GY, Kassiri Z, Jiang C, *et al.* SARS-coronavirus modulation of myocardial ACE2 expression and inflammation in patients with SARS. Eur J Clin Invest 2009; 39(7): 618-25. [http://dx.doi.org/10.1111/j.1365-2362.2009.02153.x] [PMID: 19453650]

[63] Kwong JC, Schwartz KL, Campitelli MA, *et al.* Acute myocardial infarction after laboratory-confirmed influenza infection. N Engl J Med 2018; 378(4): 345-53. [http://dx.doi.org/10.1056/NEJMoa1702090] [PMID: 29365305]

[64] Madjid M, Miller CC, Zarubaev VV, *et al.* Influenza epidemics and acute respiratory disease activity are associated with a surge in autopsy-confirmed coronary heart disease death: results from 8 years of autopsies in 34 892 subjects. Eur Heart J 2007; 28(10): 1205-10. [http://dx.doi.org/10.1093/eurheartj/ehm035] [PMID: 17440221]

[65] Chong PY, Chui P, Ling AE, *et al.* Analysis of deaths during the severe acute respiratory syndrome (SARS) epidemic in Singapore: challenges in determining a SARS diagnosis. Arch Pathol Lab Med 2004; 128(2): 195-204. [http://dx.doi.org/10.5858/2004-128-195-AODDTS] [PMID: 14736283]

[66] Bangalore S, Sharma A, Slotwiner A, *et al.* ST-segment elevation in patients with COVID-19 – a case series. N Engl J Med 2020; 382(25): 2478-80. [http://dx.doi.org/10.1056/NEJMc2009020] [PMID: 32302081]

[67] Libby P, Tabas I, Fredman G, Fisher EA. Inflammation and its resolution as determinants of acute coronary syndromes. Circ Res 2014; 114(12): 1867-79. [http://dx.doi.org/10.1161/CIRCRESAHA.114.302699] [PMID: 24902971]

[68] Bentzon JF, Otsuka F, Virmani R, Falk E. Mechanisms of plaque formation and rupture. Circ Res 2014; 114(12): 1852-66. [http://dx.doi.org/10.1161/CIRCRESAHA.114.302721] [PMID: 24902970]

[69] Varga Z, Flammer AJ, Steiger P, *et al.* Endothelial cell infection and endotheliitis in COVID-19. Lancet 2020; 395(10234): 1417-8.

[http://dx.doi.org/10.1016/S0140-6736(20)30937-5] [PMID: 32325026]

[70] Garcia S, Albaghdadi MS, Meraj PM, *et al.* Reduction in ST-segment elevation cardiac catheterization laboratory activations in the United States during COVID-19 pandemic. J Am Coll Cardiol 2020; 75(22): 2871-2.
[http://dx.doi.org/10.1016/j.jacc.2020.04.011] [PMID: 32283124]

[71] De Filippo O, D'Ascenzo F, Angelini F, *et al.* Reduced rate of hospital admissions for ACS during COVID-19 outbreak in Northern Italy. N Engl J Med 2020; 383(1): 88-9.
[http://dx.doi.org/10.1056/NEJMc2009166] [PMID: 32343497]

[72] Leor OR, Alvarez BC, Ojeda S, *et al.* Impact of the COVID-19 pandemic on interventional cardiology activity in Spain. Rec Interventional Cardiol Engl Ed REC Interv Cardiol 2020; 2(2): 82-9.

[73] De Rosa S, Spaccarotella C, Basso C, *et al.* Reduction of hospitalizations for myocardial infarction in Italy in the COVID-19 era. Eur Heart J 2020; 41(22): 2083-8.
[http://dx.doi.org/10.1093/eurheartj/ehaa409] [PMID: 32412631]

[74] Baldi E, Sechi GM, Mare C, *et al.* Out-of-hospital cardiac arrest during the COVID-19 outbreak in Italy. N Engl J Med 2020; 383(5): 496-8.
[http://dx.doi.org/10.1056/NEJMc2010418] [PMID: 32348640]

[75] Pessoa-Amorim G, Camm CF, Gajendragadkar P, *et al.* Admission of patients with STEMI since the outbreak of the COVID-19 pandemic: a survey by the European Society of Cardiology. Eur Heart J Qual Care Clin Outcomes 2020; 6(3): 210-6.
[http://dx.doi.org/10.1093/ehjqcco/qcaa046] [PMID: 32467968]

[76] Chen T, Wu D, Chen H, *et al.* Clinical characteristics of 113 deceased patients with coronavirus disease 2019: retrospective study. BMJ 2020; 368: m1091.
[http://dx.doi.org/10.1136/bmj.m1091] [PMID: 32217556]

[77] Mehra MR, Ruschitzka F. COVID-19 illness and heart failure: a missing link? JACC Heart Fail 2020; 8(6): 512-4.
[http://dx.doi.org/10.1016/j.jchf.2020.03.004] [PMID: 32360242]

[78] Dewey M, Siebes M, Kachelrieß M, *et al.* Clinical quantitative cardiac imaging for the assessment of myocardial ischaemia. Nat Rev Cardiol 2020; 17(7): 427-50.
[http://dx.doi.org/10.1038/s41569-020-0341-8] [PMID: 32094693]

[79] Manka R, Karolyi M, Polacin M, *et al.* Myocardial edema in COVID-19 on cardiac MRI. J Heart Lung Transplant 2020; 39(7): 730-2.
[http://dx.doi.org/10.1016/j.healun.2020.04.025] [PMID: 32650881]

[80] Fried JA, Ramasubbu K, Bhatt R, *et al.* The variety of cardiovascular presentations of COVID-19. Circulation 2020; 141(23): 1930-6.
[http://dx.doi.org/10.1161/CIRCULATIONAHA.120.047164] [PMID: 32243205]

[81] Prabhu SD. Cytokine-induced modulation of cardiac function. Circ Res 2004; 95(12): 1140-53.
[http://dx.doi.org/10.1161/01.RES.0000150734.79804.92] [PMID: 15591236]

[82] Liu K, Fang YY, Deng Y, *et al.* Clinical characteristics of novel coronavirus cases in tertiary hospitals in Hubei Province. Chin Med J (Engl) 2020; 133(9): 1025-31.
[http://dx.doi.org/10.1097/CM9.0000000000000744] [PMID: 32044814]

[83] Lakkireddy DR, Chung MK, Gopinathannair R, *et al.* Guidance for cardiac electrophysiology during the COVID-19 pandemic from the Heart Rhythm Society COVID-19 task force; electrophysiology section of the American College of Cardiology; and the electrocardiography and arrhythmias committee of the council on clinical cardiology, American Heart Association. Circulation 2020; 141(21): e823-31.
[http://dx.doi.org/10.1161/CIRCULATIONAHA.120.047063] [PMID: 32228309]

[84] Panigada M, Bottino N, Tagliabue P, *et al.* Hypercoagulability of COVID-19 patients in intensive care unit: A report of thromboelastography findings and other parameters of hemostasis. J Thromb

Haemost 2020; 18(7): 1738-42.
[http://dx.doi.org/10.1111/jth.14850] [PMID: 32302438]

[85] Ranucci M, Ballotta A, Di Dedda U, *et al.* The procoagulant pattern of patients with COVID-19 acute respiratory distress syndrome. J Thromb Haemost 2020; 18(7): 1747-51.
[http://dx.doi.org/10.1111/jth.14854] [PMID: 32302448]

[86] Taylor F Jr, Toh CH, Hoots K, Wada H, Levi M. Towards definition, clinical and laboratory criteria, and a scoring system for disseminated intravascular coagulation. Thromb Haemost 2001; 86(11): 1327-30.
[http://dx.doi.org/10.1055/s-0037-1616068] [PMID: 11816725]

[87] Oxley TJ, Mocco J, Majidi S, *et al.* Large-vessel stroke as a presenting feature of COVID-19 in the young. N Engl J Med 2020; 382(20): e60.
[http://dx.doi.org/10.1056/NEJMc2009787] [PMID: 32343504]

[88] Bellosta R, Luzzani L, Natalini G, *et al.* Acute limb ischemia in patients with COVID-19 pneumonia. J Vasc Surg 2020; 72(6): 1864-72.
[http://dx.doi.org/10.1016/j.jvs.2020.04.483] [PMID: 32360679]

[89] Paranjpe I, Fuster V, Lala A, *et al.* Association of treatment dose anticoagulation with in-hospital survival among hospitalized patients with COVID-19. J Am Coll Cardiol 2020; 76(1): 122-4.
[http://dx.doi.org/10.1016/j.jacc.2020.05.001] [PMID: 32387623]

[90] Tang N, Bai H, Chen X, Gong J, Li D, Sun Z. Anticoagulant treatment is associated with decreased mortality in severe coronavirus disease 2019 patients with coagulopathy. J Thromb Haemost 2020; 18(5): 1094-9.
[http://dx.doi.org/10.1111/jth.14817] [PMID: 32220112]

[91] Qiu H, Wu J, Hong L, Luo Y, Song Q, Chen D. Clinical and epidemiological features of 36 children with coronavirus disease 2019 (COVID-19) in Zhejiang, China: an observational cohort study. Lancet Infect Dis 2020; 20(6): 689-96.
[http://dx.doi.org/10.1016/S1473-3099(20)30198-5] [PMID: 32220650]

[92] Ng KW, Faulkner N, Cornish GH, *et al.* Pre-existing and *de novo* humoral immunity to SARS-CoV-2 in humans. bioRxiv 2020.
[http://dx.doi.org/10.1101/2020.05.14.095414]

[93] Chu H, Zhou J, Wong BHY, *et al.* Middle East respiratory syndrome coronavirus efficiently infects human primary T lymphocytes and activates the extrinsic and intrinsic apoptosis pathways. J Infect Dis 2016; 213(6): 904-14.
[http://dx.doi.org/10.1093/infdis/jiv380] [PMID: 26203058]

[94] Jacquelot N, Roberti MP, Enot DP, *et al.* Immunophenotyping of stage III melanoma reveals parameters associated with patient prognosis. J Invest Dermatol 2016; 136(5): 994-1001.
[http://dx.doi.org/10.1016/j.jid.2015.12.042] [PMID: 26829031]

[95] An Y, Gao S, Zhao WC, *et al.* Transforming growth factor-β and peripheral regulatory cells are negatively correlated with the overall survival of hepatocellular carcinoma. World J Gastroenterol 2018; 24(25): 2733-40.
[http://dx.doi.org/10.3748/wjg.v24.i25.2733] [PMID: 29991878]

[96] Feng P, Yan R, Dai X, Xie X, Wen H, Yang S. The alteration and clinical significance of Th1/Th2/Th17/Treg cells in patients with multiple myeloma. Inflammation 2015; 38(2): 705-9.
[http://dx.doi.org/10.1007/s10753-014-9980-4] [PMID: 25034833]

[97] Shen P, Wang A, He M, Wang Q, Zheng S. Increased circulating Lin $^{-/low}$ CD33 $^{+}$ HLA-DR $^{-}$ myeloid-derived suppressor cells in hepatocellular carcinoma patients. Hepatol Res 2014; 44(6): 639-50.
[http://dx.doi.org/10.1111/hepr.12167] [PMID: 23701406]

[98] Zitvogel L, Galluzzi L, Kepp O, Smyth MJ, Kroemer G. Type I interferons in anticancer immunity. Nat Rev Immunol 2015; 15(7): 405-14.

[http://dx.doi.org/10.1038/nri3845] [PMID: 26027717]

[99] Musella M, Manic G, De Maria R, Vitale I, Sistigu A. Type-I-interferons in infection and cancer: Unanticipated dynamics with therapeutic implications. OncoImmunology 2017; 6(5): e1314424. [http://dx.doi.org/10.1080/2162402X.2017.1314424] [PMID: 28638743]

[100] Lee AJ, Ashkar AA. The dual nature of type I and type II interferons. Front Immunol 2018; 9: 2061. [http://dx.doi.org/10.3389/fimmu.2018.02061] [PMID: 30254639]

[101] Fuertes MB, Kacha AK, Kline J, *et al.* Host type I IFN signals are required for antitumor CD^{8+} T cell responses through CD8α+ dendritic cells. J Exp Med 2011; 208(10): 2005-16. [http://dx.doi.org/10.1084/jem.20101159] [PMID: 21930765]

[102] Schreiber RD, Old LJ, Smyth MJ. Cancer immunoediting: integrating immunity's roles in cancer suppression and promotion. Science 2011; 331(6024): 1565-70. [http://dx.doi.org/10.1126/science.1203486] [PMID: 21436444]

[103] Sistigu A, Yamazaki T, Vacchelli E, *et al.* Cancer cell–autonomous contribution of type I interferon signaling to the efficacy of chemotherapy. Nat Med 2014; 20(11): 1301-9. [http://dx.doi.org/10.1038/nm.3708] [PMID: 25344738]

[104] Formenti SC, Rudqvist NP, Golden E, *et al.* Radiotherapy induces responses of lung cancer to CTLA-4 blockade. Nat Med 2018; 24(12): 1845-51. [http://dx.doi.org/10.1038/s41591-018-0232-2] [PMID: 30397353]

[105] Xue M, Fu F, Ma Y, *et al.* The PERK arm of the unfolded protein response negatively regulates transmissible gastroenteritis virus replication by suppressing protein translation and promoting type I interferon production. J Virol 2018; 92(15): e00431-18. [http://dx.doi.org/10.1128/JVI.00431-18] [PMID: 29769338]

[106] Sallard E, Lescure FX, Yazdanpanah Y, Mentre F, Peiffer-Smadja N. Type 1 interferons as a potential treatment against COVID-19. Antiviral Res 2020; 178: 104791. [http://dx.doi.org/10.1016/j.antiviral.2020.104791] [PMID: 32275914]

[107] Zhao J, Zhao J, Mangalam AK, *et al.* Airway memory CD4+ T cells mediate protective immunity against emerging respiratory coronaviruses. Immunity 2016; 44(6): 1379-91. [http://dx.doi.org/10.1016/j.immuni.2016.05.006] [PMID: 27287409]

[108] Zhao J, Wohlford-Lenane C, Zhao J, *et al.* Intranasal treatment with poly(I•C) protects aged mice from lethal respiratory virus infections. J Virol 2012; 86(21): 11416-24. [http://dx.doi.org/10.1128/JVI.01410-12] [PMID: 22915814]

[109] Kumaki Y, Salazar AM, Wandersee MK, Barnard DL. Prophylactic and therapeutic intranasal administration with an immunomodulator, Hiltonol® (Poly IC:LC), in a lethal SARS-CoV-infected BALB/c mouse model. Antiviral Res 2017; 139: 1-12. [http://dx.doi.org/10.1016/j.antiviral.2016.12.007] [PMID: 27956136]

[110] Tortura AL, Whitemore A, Agnihothram S, *et al.* Toll-like receptor 3 signaling *via* TRIF contributes to a protective innate immune response to severe acute respiratory syndrome coronavirus infection. 2015; 6: e00638-15.

[111] Blanco-Melo D, Nilsson-Payant BE, Liu WC, *et al.* Imbalanced host response to SARS-CoV-2 drives development of COVID-19. Cell 2020; 181(5): 1036-1045.e9. [http://dx.doi.org/10.1016/j.cell.2020.04.026] [PMID: 32416070]

[112] Silvin A, Chapuis N, Dunsmore G, *et al.* Elevated calprotectin and abnormal myeloid cell subsets discriminate severe from mild COVID-19. Cell 2020; 182(6): 1401-1418.e18. [http://dx.doi.org/10.1016/j.cell.2020.08.002] [PMID: 32810439]

[113] Hadjadj J, Yatim N, Barnabei L, *et al.* Impaired type I interferon activity and inflammatory responses in severe COVID-19 patients. Science 2020; 369(6504): 718-24. [http://dx.doi.org/10.1126/science.abc6027] [PMID: 32661059]

[114] Chu H, Chan JFW, Wang Y, *et al.* Comparative replication and immune activation profiles of SARS-CoV-2 and SARS-CoV in human lungs: an *ex vivo* study with implications for the pathogenesis of COVID-19. Clin Infect Dis 2020; 71(6): 1400-9. [http://dx.doi.org/10.1093/cid/ciaa410] [PMID: 32270184]

[115] Israelow B, Song E, Mao T, *et al.* Mouse model of SARS-CoV-2 reveals inflammatory role of type I interferon signaling. J Exp Med 2020; 217(12): e20201241. [http://dx.doi.org/10.1084/jem.20201241] [PMID: 32750141]

[116] Channappanavar R, Fehr AR, Zheng J, *et al.* IFN-I response timing relative to virus replication determines MERS coronavirus infection outcomes. J Clin Invest 2019; 129(9): 3625-39. [http://dx.doi.org/10.1172/JCI126363] [PMID: 31355779]

[117] Channappanavar R, Fehr AR, Vijay R, *et al.* Dysregulated type I interferon and inflammatory monocyte-macrophage responses cause lethal pneumonia in SARS-CoV-infected mice. Cell Host Microbe 2016; 19(2): 181-93. [http://dx.doi.org/10.1016/j.chom.2016.01.007] [PMID: 26867177]

[118] Jacquelot N, Yamazaki T, Roberti MP, *et al.* Sustained Type I interferon signaling as a mechanism of resistance to PD-1 blockade. Cell Res 2019; 29(10): 846-61. [http://dx.doi.org/10.1038/s41422-019-0224-x] [PMID: 31481761]

[119] Bravo-Jaimes K, Marcellon R, Varanitskaya L, *et al.* Opportunities for improved cardiovascular disease prevention in oncology patients. Curr Opin Cardiol 2020; 35(5): 531-7. [http://dx.doi.org/10.1097/HCO.0000000000000767] [PMID: 32649353]

[120] Tini G, Sarocchi M, Tocci G, *et al.* Arterial hypertension in cancer: The elephant in the room. Int J Cardiol 2019; 281: 133-9. [http://dx.doi.org/10.1016/j.ijcard.2019.01.082] [PMID: 30718135]

[121] Essa H, Pettitt AR, Lip GYH. Hypertension and cardiovascular risk factors when treating cancer patients: underrecognised and undertreated. J Hum Hypertens 2020; 946-64. [PMID: 32788664]

[122] Tavakkoli M, Wilkins CR, Mones JV, Mauro MJ. A novel paradigm between leukocytosis, G-CSF secretion, neutrophil-to-lymphocyte ratio, myeloid-derived suppressor cells, and prognosis in non-small cell lung cancer. Front Oncol 2019; 9: 295. [http://dx.doi.org/10.3389/fonc.2019.00295] [PMID: 31080780]

[123] Jin H, Yoo Y, Kim Y, Kim Y, Cho J, Lee YS. Radiation-induced lung fibrosis: preclinical animal models and therapeutic strategies. Cancers (Basel) 2020; 12(6): 1561. [http://dx.doi.org/10.3390/cancers12061561] [PMID: 32545674]

[124] Addeo A, Obeid M, Friedlaender A. COVID-19 and lung cancer: risks, mechanisms and treatment interactions. J Immunother Cancer 2020; 8(1): e000892. [http://dx.doi.org/10.1136/jitc-2020-000892] [PMID: 32434788]

CHAPTER 5

Indian Expedition against Covid-19 through Traditional Drugs

Rupesh Kumar Pandey[1], **Sokindra Kumar**[1], **Lubhan Singh**[1], **Priyanka Pandey**[2], **Rakesh Sagar**[3], **Ravindra Kumar Pandey**[4] and **Shiv Shankar Shukla**[4,*]

[1] *KSCP, Swami Vivekanand Subharti University, Meerut, Uttar Pradesh, India*

[2] *Swami Vivekanand College of Pharmacy, Indore, Madhya Pradesh, India*

[3] *Department of Pharmacy, SGSITS Campus Indore, Madhya Pradesh, India*

[4] *Columbia Institute of Pharmacy, Tekari, Raipur, Chhattisgarh, India*

Abstract: COVID-19 was a menace to India's densely populated country. The entire globe is dealing with the same problem, but India is fighting it in its own unique way, namely *via* the use of ancient traditional medicines. Every country used to shut down as a first line of defence to safeguard its population; the whole globe came to a halt during the epidemic, and people were confined to their homes. A preparation program was needed to prepare their country and reconstruct their medical institution in the event of a pandemic. The entire globe is paying tribute to all of the corona warriors for their selfless commitment and unwavering care for patients during this critical period. The Indian government has also taken some swift moves to combat the sickness by employing certain traditional medicines. Many researchers went to considerable lengths not just to give therapy but also preventative strategies. Immunity has been proven to be the most critical factor in the illness. This chapter tries to highlight the most important traditional medications utilised by Indians from ancient times. Indians employ a variety of spices in their cooking, many of which are high in chemical elements that can help with a variety of ailments. When Ayurveda has been called upon, it has demonstrated its usefulness several times. The usage of traditional medications in every home is well documented in the Indian system. Since ancient times, the customary approach has been shown to be reliable and applicable. Many ailments have been categorised and evidence-based information has been provided by Indian literature such as the Ayurvedic Pharmacopeia and Chark Samhita. It also reflected the immunity level of Indians and they explored the uses of these traditional drugs in the dosage form *i.e.* kadha, Chwanpras, *etc.* The expedition showed great reflection in terms of the recovery rate of patients *i.e.* 97.15 percent, deaths were also minimized as compared to developed countries in terms of the population ratio.

* **Corresponding author Shiv Shankar Shukla:** Department of Pharmaceutics Columbia Institute of Pharmacy, Tekari Raipur Chhattisgarh, India; Tel: 91-9479347077; E-mail: shivpharma007@gmail.com

Keywords: Ayurveda, Chark Samhita, Immunity, Traditional drugs.

1. INTRODUCTION

COVID-19 has not only affected the people but it deteriorated the economic conditions of countries too. Globally many people lost their jobs due to lockdown but that was the need of the hour. We will not forget this pandemic time and it would be a black chapter in history. People were locked down in their houses and they were in a fearful state while being in social gatherings. During this pandemic, students were silent and educational institutes closed. The disease started in Wuhan China in December 2019 and spread globally within a short period. Nobody has the answer to the treatment's concern; every country was looking for its best scientific efforts. India a religious country with a huge population started its expedition for COVID-19 in its traditional way. Indian people use many herbal drugs on day to day basis. While writing this book, it is a matter of pleasure that a huge vaccination program is running in India. India is also amongst those countries that are manufacturing vaccines for the whole world.

Indian government started some new programs to strengthen the health facilities in many COVID-19 hospital setups in each district. The aim was to maximize the testing protocols, for that many labs were established specifically for COVID-19 testing, and today India is testing approx 10 lacks cases daily through these labs. The self-reliant program is also running for the health care segment also. Many startup programs have also been initiated which are playing an important role in building the economy as well as improving the patient's status.

1.1. Disease Etiology

Corona virus is an enveloped and single-stranded RNA virus. They are zoonotic in nature and can transmit from animals to humans. They are largely classified as alpha, Beta, Gama, and Delta Corona virus with their different genomic structures. Some research suggests that alpha and Beta Corona virus cause infection only in mammals. Human Coronaviruses such as 229E and NL63 are responsible for common cold and cough and belong to α Corona virus. Hemagglutinin esterase is a glycoprotein that helps viruses with attack mechanisms. Several coronaviruses do have envelope-associated hemagglutinin-esterase protein (HE), which helps in the attachment and destruction of certain sialic acid receptors that are found on the host cell surface.

Coronavirus contains a spike protein that has a multifunctional molecular machinery that helps in Coronavirus entry into host cells. Based on a structural study, it has been revealed that the mechanism is based on binding to the receptor on the host cell surface through its S1 subunit and then through the S2 subunit, it fuses viral and host membranes.

1.2. Regulation of Spike Protein

The life cycle of the virus and, host consists of these steps *i.e.* attachment to the site, penetration, biosynthesis, growth, and release. When binding occurs to the host receptor, it moves inside the host cells through endocytosis or by membrane fusion thereby starting replication. The viral mRNA plays an important role in the biosynthesis of viral proteins which mature and are released. Structural studies suggest that corona viruses have a spike (S), membrane (M), envelope (E), and nucleocapsid (N). Spike has a transmembrane glycoprotein that protrudes to the viral surface and shows multiplicity of Corona virus. There are two functional subunits *i.e.* S1 subunit which has the binding ability to the host cell receptor where S2 subunit is for penetration of the viral cellular membranes, according to some previous research work Angiotensin-converting enzyme 2 identified as a regulating receptor for SARS-Cov [1]. Studies based on structure and function implicated that these spike proteins bind to ACE2 [2 - 4]. These ACE2 are mostly found in the lungs where they play an important role in the disease.

1.3. Indian Traditional Drugs

India is linked with the use of traditional medicine since ancient times. The basic knowledge of these systems gained through literature can be seen in each household. Indian traditional medicinal system is unique and the oldest in the world.

Traditional systems of medicines played a crucial role in the development of the global healthcare system. Traditional medicine is useful in diverse health-related practices and approaches, divine knowledge, skills, and practices related to plants, and minerals. Indian civilization is wide-ranging having versatile cultural aspects and is one of the oldest for mankind. Indian traditional medicinal system is one of the oldest traditional medicinal systems in the world. India has distinctive characteristics and well-acclaimed traditional systems of medicine *i.e.* Ayurveda, Unani, Siddha, Yoga, naturopathy, and homeopathy, however, homeopathy is not an indigenous system and came into existence in India in the eighteenth century, it completely integrated into the Indian civilization and got improved like any other traditional medicinal system and it is believed as part of Indian Systems of Medicine. The unani system originated in Greece, and later it was introduced in India by Arabs.

Tribal medicines are a new segment apart from other systems which need to be explored more. These are also important for the indigenous healthcare system, though they have not been prearranged under any category. The classical transcripts of the Indian traditional medicine system Ayurveda include Rigveda, Atharvaveda, Charaka Samhita, and Sushruta Samhita.

2. INDIAN HERBAL FORMULATIONS USED AS IMMUNITY BOOSTER FOR COVID-19

Many herbal formulations were used by Indian people during the pandemic. We aim to highlight some drugs which contain bioactive compounds and play an important role in fighting the disease. As rightly said, prevention is better than cure, Indian people strengthen their immunity through available traditional medicines.

2.1. *Alium Sativum*

The herb is extensively used by Indian people on day to day basis for food preparation methods. Lahsun is the common name and every household uses it since ancient times. *Allium sativum*, Family: Amaryllidaceae is the herb that is used very commonly in India.

Chemical constituents- allicin, ajones, allyl methyl thiosulfinate, methyl allyl thiosulfinate, Diallyl sulfide (DAS), Diallyl disulfide, Diallyl trisulfide, Allyl methyl sulfide,2-Vinyl-4H-1,3-dithiin.

Bioactive compounds present in *alium sativam* and their pharmacological activities

The presence of bioactive compound shows great pharmacological activities we aim to highlight the pharmacological activities that can explain the efficacy of drugs against COVID-19.

S. No	Bioactive Compounds	Pharmacological Activity	Reference
1.	Allicin, Diallyl trisulfide	Antiviral	[5]
2.	Diallyl disulfide, Diallyl trisulfide	Antifungal	[6]
3.	Allicin	Antibacterial Activity	[7]
4.	Diallyl trisulfide, Allicin, ajones	Anti-Protozoal	[5]
5.	Allin,allicin, Diallyl disulfide, Diallyl trisulfide, Diallyl sulfide	Antioxidant	[7-9]
6.	Allicin, Diallyl sulfide, Thiacremonone	Anti-Inflammatory	[10-12]

cont.....

S. No	Bioactive Compounds	Pharmacological Activity	Reference
7.	Allicin	Immunomodulatory	[13]

2.2. *Ocimum Sanctum*

Popularly known as 'tulsi' in the Hindi language, the plant is worshiped by Indian people as holy basil; the plant has huge medicinal value. It's used in many preparations; the plant also has air purification ability, generally planted in a yard of houses. The major chemical constituents present in Tulsi are saponins, triterpenoids, flavonoids and tannins, Rosmarinic acid, apigenin, cirsimaritin, and isothymonin.

Bioactive compounds present in *ocimum sanctum* and their pharmacological activities

S. No	Bioactive Compounds	Pharmacological Activity	Reference
1.	Eugenol	Antiviral	[14, 15]
2.	Eugenol	Cough and Sore Throat	[16]
3.	Fixed oil	Antipyretic activity	[17]
4.	Orientin and vicenin	Immunomodulatory activity, anti oxidant	[18]
5.	Linoleic acid	Antimicrobial activity	[19]

2.3. *Cinnamomum Verum*

It's known as Dalchini in the Hindi language. Cinnamon contains chemical constituents such as cinnamaldehyde, cinnamate, cinnamic acid, and numerous essential oils *trans*-cinnamaldehyde, cinnamyl acetate, eugenol, L-borneol, caryophyllene oxide, b-caryophyllene, L-bornyl acetate, E-nerolidol, α-cubebene, α-terpineol, terpinolene, and α-thujene.

Bioactive compounds present in *Cinnamomum verum* and their pharmacological activities.

S. No	Bioactive Compounds	Pharmacological Activity	Reference
1.	Cinnamaldehyde	Antimicrobial activity	[20]
2.	Linalyl acetate	Anti allergic	[21]
3.	Terpinenes	Antiviral	[22]
4.	Carboxylic acid	Antioxidant	[23]
5.	Eugenol	Anti-inflammatory	[24]
6.	Sapogenin, Alkaloids	Analgesic	[25]

2.4. *Acacia Arabica*

Acacia arabica is a plant known as babool in Hindi. The major chemical constituents are tannin, stearic acid, kaempferol-3- glucoside, isoquercetin, leucocyanidin with polyphenolic compounds (+) dicatechin, quercetin, gallic acid and ∞ - amyrin, ß-sitosterol.

Bioactive compounds present in *Acacia arabica* and their pharmacological activities

S. No	Bioactive Compounds	Pharmacological Activity	Reference
1.	Alkaloids, tannins and glycosides	Antimicrobial activity	[26, 27]
2.	Tannins	Antioxidant	[28]
3.	Phenolic compounds	Anti-inflammatory effects	[29]
4.	Polyphenolic compounds	Antiviral	[30]

2.5. *Azadirachta Indica*

Azadirachta indica L. in Hindi known as Neem has a great therapeutic role in health care management due to being a rich source of various types of ingredients, such as various active constituents like azadirachtin, nimbolinin, nimbin, nimbidin, nimbidol, sodium nimbinate, gedunin, salannin, and quercetin. The leaf part contains some important ingredients nimbin, nimbanene, 6-desacetylnimbinene, nimbandiol, nimbolide, ascorbic acid, n-hexacosanol, and amino acid, 7-desacetyl-7-benzoylazadiradione, 7-desacetyl-7-benzoylgedunin, 17-hydroxyazadiradione, and nimbiol.

Bioactive compounds present in *Azadirachta indica* and their pharmacological activities

S. No	Bioactive Compounds	Pharmacological Activity	References
1.	Flavonoids, Triterpenoids	Anti viral	[31]
2.	Nimbidin	Antibacterial	[32]
3.	Polysaccharides G2A, G3A	Anti-inflammatory	[33]
4.	NB-2 Peptidoglucan	Immunomodulatory	[34]

2.6. *Citrus Limon*

The plant is known as neebu in Hindi. The fruit is used by Indian people in many ways. Various chemical constituents are present in *Citrus limon* fruit and its juice which correlate its usefulness in many diseases. Flavonoids such as eriodictyol, hesperidin, hesperetin, naringin; flavones *i.e.* apigenin, diosmin, quercetin; and their derivatives: flavonols like limocitrin and spinacetin, orientin and vitexin and also other flavonoids are additionally detected. *Citrus limon* has the highest content of eriocitrin. Phenolic acids are another important group of compounds found both in the juice and fruit1. There are mainly two such compounds in the juice—ferulic acid and synapic acid, and their derivatives. In the fruit, there are also carboxylic acids, carbohydrates, amino acids, a complex of vitamins B, predominantly vitamin C.

Bioactive compounds present in *Citrus limon* and their pharmacological activities

S. No	Bioactive Compounds	Pharmacological Activity	Reference
1.	Hesperidin and Hesperetin	Antioxidant Activity	[35, 36]
2.	D-limonene	Anti-Inflammatory Activity	[37, 38]
3.	D-limonene, β-pinene, citral	Antimicrobial Activity	[39, 40]
4.	Essential oil	Antiviral Activity	[41, 42]

2.7. *Zinger Oficinale*

Ginger is known as adrak in Hindi having many active constituents like terpene and phenolic compounds mainly gingerols, shogaols, and paradols. In fresh ginger, gingerols are the major polyphenols, such as 6-gingerol, 8-gingerol, and 10-gingerol. There are also many other phenolic compounds in ginger, such as quercetin, zingerone, gingerenone-A, and 6-dehydrogingerdione . Moreover, there are several terpene components in ginger, such as β-bisabolene, α-curcumene, zingiberene, α-farnesene, and β-sesquiphellandrene, which are considered to be the main constituents of ginger essential oils.

Bioactive compounds of *Zinger oficinale* and their pharmacological activities

S. No	Bioactive Compounds	Pharmacological Activity	Reference
1.	6-shogaol	antioxidant activity	[43]
2.	essential oil	Antimicrobial activity	[44]
3.	Zingerone	Anti-inflammatory	[45]

2.8. *Curcuma Longa*

It is known as Haldi in Hindi, having great importance in the Hindu religion. During this pandemic time, Indian people are using this in many perpetrations. It has many important chemical constituents such as Curcumin, Bis-desmethoxycurcumin, Desmethoxy Curcumin, Tetrahydro Curcumin, Alpha Curcumene, Ar- turmerone, Curcumol, Curdione, Dehydro Curdione, and Zingiberene.

Bioactive compounds present in *Curcuma longa* and their pharmacological activities

S. No	Bioactive Compounds	Pharmacological Activity	Reference
1.	Curcumin	Antiviral, Antioxidant, Anti-EBV, Immunostimulant	[46]
2.	Bis-desmethoxycurcumin	Antiiflammatory	[46]
3.	Tetrahydro Curcumin	Antioxidant, Antiinflammatory	[46]
4.	Zingiberene	Antirhinoviral,	[46]
5.	DehydroCurdione	Analgesic, Antipyretic,	[46]

2.9. Plant Metabolite Potential as Immunity Booster for Covid -19

2.9.1. Flavonoids

Flavonoids have antiviral therapeutic potential. A study suggests more than a thousand different compounds to be present in them [47]. These metabolites are considered as one of the most abundantly present polyphenols in our diet and are generally found as glycosides and acylglycosides in vegetables and fruits. Many flavonoids are present naturally in plants including quercetin, naringin, hesperetin, catechin, and have proven their activity against the plethora of animal viruses such as HSV-1, respiratory syncytial virus, parainfluenza virus type 3, and polio-virus type 1 [48].

Some researchers reported the anti-viral activity of flavonoids earlier, against severe acute respiratory syndrome coronavirus (SARS-CoV) [49]. The mechanism of action is based on the inhibition of cellular receptor kinases including MAPKs, the serine/threonine-specific protein kinase (Akt), and the phosphatidylinositol-4,5-bisphosphate 3-kinase (PI3-K) and as consequence interferes with the cellular signal transduction cascades by which they suppress the viral infection [50].

2.9.2. Polyphenols

Polyphenols display a wide range of biological activities and are known to increase immune response to cells to foreign infestations and in response permit the cellular accumulation of different types of polyphenols through varied receptors, which trigger signaling pathways and initiate immune responses [51]. The recent *in-silico* study suggests that natural polyphenols can be used as potent COVID-19 protease (Mpro) inhibitors [52]. The study was carried by using the molecular docking technique. The virus COVID-19 was docked with 80 different flavonoids and the results indicated that compounds such as rutin, apiin, hesperidin, diosmin, and diacetylcurcumin, *etc*. had an effective inhibitory effect on protease enzyme and they might have a role in lowering the symptoms of COVID-19 infection.

2.9.3. Terpenoids

The triterpenes have 6 isoprene units with squalene as a prototype and are diversely found in plant species [53]. They have an important role in the modulation of cellular metabolism, specifically the biosynthesis of sterols and have a significant level of antiviral activity [54].

Various research work suggests that they affect HSV1 and HSV2. These include dammaradienol, dammarenediol-II, dammarenolic acid, hydroxyhopanone, hydroxydammarenone-I, shoreic acid, ursonic acid, hydroxyoleanonic lactone, and eichlerianic acid [55]. Structurally coronavirus is composed of a single-stranded RNA, reported to be one of the longest RNA viruses. This RNA strand acts as an RNA messenger, when it transmits into a cell, it stimulates the synthesis of two polyproteins which are further composed of novel replication and transmission complexes that regulate the synthesis of RNA, structural proteins and enhance the activity of protease enzymes. Here protease enzyme has significant participation in the fragmentation of the polyprotein [56, 57]. Apart from designing and chemical synthesis of protease inhibitors, one of the most recent therapeutic strategies to cure viral infection is to identify the inhibitors of these enzymes in natural products and compounds.

2.9.4. Dipeptides

The dipeptides can be a good drug candidate for COVID-19 as it has an activity similar to protease and is an approved target.

3. SCOPE, CHALLENGES AND POTENTIAL SOLUTION

The traditional medicine system is one of the oldest forms of health care in the world. It's used in the prevention as well as treatment of many diseases. The traditional medicine system is also known as complementary and alternative, or ethnic medicine, it still plays a key role in many countries today. Traditional medicines are mostly derived from natural products.

We have seen Traditional drugs that are well accepted by people nowadays and the reason behind this is the least adverse effect and good therapeutic efficacy. Many pharmaceutical companies are coming into the market and getting good business. Every country is rich with fauna and flora which have some therapeutic values. It should also be noted that these drugs are easily available and used on a day to day basis by people. The uniqueness of these medicines is that they not only cure one disease but have some other activities too. Recent approaches of researchers also show great interest in the traditional system drug discovery process. The adverse effects are also increasing with the allopathic medication which is a great concern in front of the world so here is the time to explore a therapy which is safe for the patient. Indian people use this medication system since the old times with some important herbs which are used for different diseases.

3.1. Challenges

The present scenario shows the awareness and general acceptability of the use of herbal drugs that is increasing day by day in medical practice. It should be noted that the majority of the world's population depends on herbal medicines and products for healthy living. This increase in the use of herbal products has also given rise to various forms of adulteration and abuse of the products leading to consumers' and manufacturers' disappointment. The challenge in front of us is huge which is making the global herbal market unsafe.

3.2. Potential Solution

For standardization and quality control of herbal crude drugs –WHO (1996a and b, 1992) has given guidelines for standardization and quality control of herbals. This process involves the physicochemical evaluation of crude drugs covering features like selection and handling of crude materials, safety, efficacy, and stability assessment of the finished product, documentation of safety and risk based on experience, provision of product information to the consumer, and product promotion.

- **Macro and microscopic examination**: for identification of right variety and adulterants.
- **Presence of foreign organic matter**: that involves the removal of matter other than source plant to get the drug in the pure form.
- **Calculation of ash values**: for purity of crude drug – total ash, sulphated ash, water-soluble ash, and acid insoluble ash, *etc*.
- **Presence of moisture content**: determination of moisture content helps to reduce errors in the estimation of the actual weight of drug material *i.e.* low moisture suggests better stability against degradation of the product.

- **Extractive values**: these are indicative weights of the extractable chemical constituents of the crude drug under different solvents environments.
- **Crude fiber**: this helps to determine the woody material component, and it is a criterion for judging purity.
- **Qualitative chemical evaluation**: identification and characterization of a crude drug concerning phytochemicals. It is a different analytical technique to detect and isolate the active constituents. Phytochemical screening techniques entail botanical identification, extraction with suitable solvents, purification, and characterization of the active constituents of pharmaceutical significance.
- **Chromatographic examination**: includes detection of crude drug based on the use of major chemical constituents as markers.
- **Quantitative chemical evaluation**: to estimate the amount of the major classes of constituents.
- **Toxicological studies**: identification of the toxic residues, potentially toxic elements, safety studies in animals like LD50, and Microbial assay to establish the absence or presence of potentially harmful microorganisms. The processes mentioned for a wide collection of scientific investigations, which include physical, chemical, and biological evaluation employing various analytical methods and tools. The precise aims of these investigations in assuring herbal quality are as varied as the processes employed.

Standardization is one of the important parameters needed for the use of herbal drugs. Many kinds of literature are available for the use of herbal drugs but the problem is to prove the same through standardization parameters. Some problems may arise if a person using these drugs is not aware of the therapeutic dosage of these drugs. More work is to be needed in the standardization part of these medications.

4. FUTURE PROSPECTS

Due to the ongoing Pandemic COVID-19, the need is to discover alternative medicines. Herbal Medicines Are Time Tested Drugs since Ancient Time. Many Herbal drugs have proven their efficacy against viral diseases in the past. The presence of various primary and secondary metabolites can be a good option for targeting the virus *i.e.* penetration, replication, expression, and invasion part. We have seen the plants and their metabolites that prove their efficacy by increasing the immunity which not only prevented the disease but cured it. Today we have only *in vitro* data that shows the efficacy of these drugs in covid19, so there is a need to establish the same *in vivo* method through which we can get some direction for drug discovery process for the Pandemic COVID19.

CONCLUSION

The plant, as one of the important sources, still maintains its original place in the treatment of various diseases with minimum side effects [58]. The aim of this chapter is to transform the knowledge of traditional drugs in other countries too. The pandemic is continued, and this work can give some directions to the world for future research. Indian people are using these drugs in this COVID-19 and believe them to be prophylactic medication. We focused on these medications and correlated them with the available scientific-based work which strengthens the present work. The different country guidelines are there to fight with the pandemic. Everybody should follow the same, stay safe and stay healthy.

CONSENT FOR PUBLICATION

Not applicable.

CONFLICT OF INTEREST

The author declares no conflict of interest, financial or otherwise.

ACKNOWLEDGEMENTS

Declared none.

REFERENCES

[1] Li W, Moore MJ, Vasilieva N, *et al.* Angiotensin-converting enzyme 2 is a functional receptor for the SARS coronavirus. Nature 2003; 426(6965): 450-4. [http://dx.doi.org/10.1038/nature02145] [PMID: 14647384]

[2] Chen Y, Guo Y, Pan Y, Zhao ZJ. Structure analysis of the receptor binding of 2019-nCoV. Biochem Biophys Res Commun 2020; 525(1): 135-40. Epub ahead of print [http://dx.doi.org/10.1016/j.bbrc.2020.02.071] [PMID: 32081428]

[3] Walls AC, Park YJ, Tortorici MA, Wall A, McGuire AT, Veesler D. Structure, function, and antigenicity of the SARS-CoV-2 spike glycoprotein. Cell 2020; 181(2): 281-292.e6. [http://dx.doi.org/10.1016/j.cell.2020.02.058] [PMID: 32155444]

[4] Letko M, Marzi A, Munster V. Functional assessment of cell entry and receptor usage for SARS-Co--2 and other lineage B betacoronaviruses. Nat Microbiol 2020; 5(4): 562-9. [http://dx.doi.org/10.1038/s41564-020-0688-y] [PMID: 32094589]

[5] Zhen H, Fang F, Ye D, *et al.* Experimental study on the action of allitridin against human cytomegalovirus *in vitro*: Inhibitory effects on immediate-early genes. Antiviral Res 2006; 72(1): 68-74. [http://dx.doi.org/10.1016/j.antiviral.2006.03.017] [PMID: 16844239]

[6] Kuda T, Iwai A, Yano T. Effect of red pepper *Capsicum annuum* var. conoides and garlic *Allium sativum* on plasma lipid levels and cecal microflora in mice fed beef tallow. Food Chem Toxicol 2004; 42(10): 1695-700. [http://dx.doi.org/10.1016/j.fct.2004.06.007] [PMID: 15354321]

[7] Gruhlke MC, Nwachwukwu I, Arbach M, Anwar A, Noll U, Slusarenko AJ. Allicin from garlic,

effective in controlling several plant diseases, is a reactive sulfur species (RSS) that pushes cells into apoptosis; Proceedings of the Modern fungicides and antifungal compounds VI. 16th International Reinhardsbrunn Symposium Friedrichroda, Germany. 2010.2010.

[8] Shang A, Cao SY, Xu XY, *et al.* Bioactive compounds and biological functions of garlic (*Allium sativum* L.). Foods 2019; 8(7): 246.
[http://dx.doi.org/10.3390/foods8070246] [PMID: 31284512]

[9] Abdel-Hafeez EH, Ahmad AK, Kamal AM, Abdellatif MZM, Abdelgelil NH. *In vivo* antiprotozoan effects of garlic (*Allium sativum*) and ginger (*Zingiber officinale*) extracts on experimentally infected mice with Blastocystis spp. Parasitol Res 2015; 114(9): 3439-44.
[http://dx.doi.org/10.1007/s00436-015-4569-x] [PMID: 26085068]

[10] Abdel-Daim MM, Abushouk AI, Bungău SG, *et al.* Protective effects of thymoquinone and diallyl sulphide against malathion-induced toxicity in rats. Environ Sci Pollut Res Int 2020; 27(10): 10228-35.
[http://dx.doi.org/10.1007/s11356-019-07580-y] [PMID: 31933077]

[11] Jin P, Kim JA, Choi DY, Lee YJ, Jung HS, Hong JT. Anti-inflammatory and anti-amyloidogenic effects of a small molecule, 2,4-bis(p-hydroxyphenyl)-2-butenal in Tg2576 Alzheimer's disease mice model. J Neuroinflammation 2013; 10(1): 767.
[http://dx.doi.org/10.1186/1742-2094-10-2] [PMID: 23289709]

[12] Bayan L, Koulivand PH, Gorji A. Garlic: a review of potential therapeutic effects. Avicenna J Phytomed 2014; 4(1): 1-14.
[PMID: 25050296]

[13] Liu SG, Ren PY, Wang GY, Yao SX, He XJ. Allicin protects spinal cord neurons from glutamate-induced oxidative stress through regulating the heat shock protein 70/inducible nitric oxide synthase pathway. Food Funct 2015; 6(1): 320-9.
[http://dx.doi.org/10.1039/C4FO00761A] [PMID: 25473931]

[14] Mishra P, Mishra S. Study of antibacterial activity of Ocimum sanctum extract against gram positive and gram negative bacteria. 2011.
[http://dx.doi.org/10.3923/ajft.2011.336.341]

[15] Farivar TN, Fard AHM, Zahedani SS, Naderi M, Moud BS. Anti tuberculosis effect of Ocimum sanctum extracts in *in-vitro* and macrophage culture. J Medicinal Sci 2006; 6: 348-51.

[16] Singh S, Agrwal SS. anti asthmatic and anti inflammatory activity of ocimum sanctum. Int J Pharmacol 1991; 29: 306.

[17] Singh S, Taneja M, Majumdar DK. Biological activities of Ocimum sanctum L. fixed oil--an overview. Indian J Exp Biol 2007; 45(5): 403-12.
[PMID: 17569280]

[18] Kelm MA, Nair MG, Strasburg GM, DeWitt DL. Antioxidant and cyclooxygenase inhibitory phenolic compounds from Ocimum sanctum Linn. Phytomedicine 2000; 7(1): 7-13.
[http://dx.doi.org/10.1016/S0944-7113(00)80015-X] [PMID: 10782484]

[19] Rahman MS, Khan MMH, Jamal MAHM. Antibacterial. Anti-bactirial evaluation and minimum inhibitory concentration analysis of Oxalis corniculata and Ocimum sanctum against bacterial pathogens. Biotechonology 2010; 9: 533-6.

[20] Ali NAM, Mohtar M, Shaari K, Rahmanii M, Ali AM, Jantan IB. Chemical composition and antimicrobial activities of the essential oils of *Cinnamomum aureofulvum* Gamb. J Essent Oil Res 2002; 14(2): 135-8.
[http://dx.doi.org/10.1080/10412905.2002.9699798]

[21] Insung A, Pumnuan J, Mahakittikun V, Wangapai T. Effectiveness of essential oils of medicinal plants at reducing the amounts of allergen produced by the European house dust mite, <i>Dermatophagoides pteronyssinus</i> (Trouessart). Nihon Dani Gakkaishi 2016; 25 (Suppl. 1): S179-84.

[http://dx.doi.org/10.2300/acari.25.Suppl_179]

[22] Lin CC, Cheng HY, Fang BJ. Anti-herpes virus type 2 activity of herbal medicines from Taiwan. Pharm Biol 2003; 41(4): 259-62.
[http://dx.doi.org/10.1076/phbi.41.4.259.15676]

[23] Salleh WMNHW, Ahmad F, Yen KH. Evaluation of antioxidant, anticholinesterase and antityrosinase activities of Malaysian *Cinnamomum* species. Dhaka University Journal of Pharmaceutical Sciences 2016; 14(2): 125-32.
[http://dx.doi.org/10.3329/dujps.v14i2.28500]

[24] Sumiwi SA, Subarnas A, Supriyatna S, Abdasah M, Muchtaridi M. Analysis of chemical composition and its analgesic and anti-inflammatory activity of essential oil of sintoc bark (Cinnamomum sintoc bl.) using *in vivo* methods. J Appl Pharm Sci 2015; 5: 058-6%.

[25] Torres RC, Sison FM, Ysrael MC. Phytochemical screening and biological studies on the crude methanol extract of *Cinnamomum* mercadoi Vidal. Philipp J Sci 2003; 132: 27-32.

[26] Deshpande SN. Preliminary Phytochemical Analysis and *in vitro* investigation of antibacterial activity of Acacia nilotica against clinical isolates. J Pharmacogn Phytochem 2013; 1(5): 23-7.

[27] Banso A. Phytochemical and antibacterial investigation of bark extracts of Acacia nilotica. 2009.

[28] Sadiq MB, Hanpithakpong W, Tarning J, Anal AK. Screening of phytochemicals and *in vitro* evaluation of antibacterial and antioxidant activities of leaves, pods and bark extracts of Acacia nilotica (L.) Del. Ind Crops Prod 2015; 77: 873-82.
[http://dx.doi.org/10.1016/j.indcrop.2015.09.067]

[29] Huang WY, Cai YZ, Zhang Y. Natural phenolic compounds from medicinal herbs and dietary plants: potential use for cancer prevention. Nutr Cancer 2009; 62(1): 1-20.
[http://dx.doi.org/10.1080/01635580903191585] [PMID: 20043255]

[30] Hussein G, Miyashiro H, Nakamura N, *et al.* Inhibitory effects of Sudanese plant extracts on HCV-1 replication and HCV-1 protease. Phytotherapy resrech 1999; 13(1): 31-6.

[31] Uzzaman S. Pharmacological activities of neem (Azadirachta indica): A review. International Journal of Pharmacognosy and Life Science 2020; 1(1): 38-41.
[http://dx.doi.org/10.33545/27072827.2020.v1.i1a.8]

[32] Murthy PS, Sirsi M. Pharmacological studies on Melia azadirachta, Linn. (n. o. Meliaceae). Indian J Psychol 1958; 2(2): 387-96.
[PMID: 13562911]

[33] Fujiwara T, Sugishita E, Takeda T, *et al.* Further studies on the structure of polysaccharides from the bark of Melia azadirachta. Chem Pharm Bull (Tokyo) 1984; 32(4): 1385-91.
[http://dx.doi.org/10.1248/cpb.32.1385]

[34] van der Nat JM, Klerx JPAM, van Dijk H, De Silva KTD, Labadie RP. Immunomodulatory activity of an aqueous extract of Azadirachta indica stem bark. J Ethnopharmacol 1987; 19(2): 125-31.
[http://dx.doi.org/10.1016/0378-8741(87)90036-5] [PMID: 3302545]

[35] Robards K, Antolovich M. Analytical chemistry of fruit bioflavonoids. A review. Analyst (Lond) 1997; 122(2): 11R-34R.
[http://dx.doi.org/10.1039/a606499j]

[36] Parhiz H, Roohbakhsh A, Soltani F, Rezaee R, Iranshahi M. Antioxidant and anti-inflammatory properties of the citrus flavonoids hesperidin and hesperetin: an updated review of their molecular mechanisms and experimental models. Phytother Res 2015; 29(3): 323-31.
[http://dx.doi.org/10.1002/ptr.5256] [PMID: 25394264]

[37] Xavier SM, Barbosa CO, Barros DO, Silva RF, Oliveira AA, Freitas RM. Vitamin C antioxidant effects in hippocampus of adult Wistar rats after seizures and status epilepticus induced by pilocarpine. Neurosci Lett 2007; 420(1): 76-9.

[http://dx.doi.org/10.1016/j.neulet.2007.04.056] [PMID: 17512118]

[38] Amorim JL, Simas DLR, Pinheiro MMG, *et al.* Anti-inflammatory properties and chemical characterization of the essential oils of four *Citrus* species. PLoS One 2016; 11(4): e0153643. [http://dx.doi.org/10.1371/journal.pone.0153643] [PMID: 27088973]

[39] Hamdan D, Ashour ML, Mulyaningsih S, El-Shazly A, Wink M. Chemical composition of the essential oils of variegated pink-fleshed lemon (*Citrus* x *limon* L. Burm. f.) and their anti-inflammatory and antimicrobial activities. Zeitschrift fur Naturforsch.-Sect. C J Biosci 2013; 68C: 275-84.

[40] Bhatia H, Pal Sharma Y, Manhas RK, Kumar K. Traditional phytoremedies for the treatment of menstrual disorders in district Udhampur, J&K, India. J Ethnopharmacol 2015; 160: 202-10. [http://dx.doi.org/10.1016/j.jep.2014.11.041] [PMID: 25479156]

[41] Otang WM, Afolayan AJ. Antimicrobial and antioxidant efficacy of *Citrus limon* L. peel extracts used for skin diseases by Xhosa tribe of Amathole District, Eastern Cape, South Africa. S Afr J Bot 2016; 102: 46-9.
[http://dx.doi.org/10.1016/j.sajb.2015.08.005]

[42] Minami M, Kita M, Nakaya T, Yamamoto T, Kuriyama H, Imanishi J. The inhibitory effect of essential oils on herpes simplex virus type-1 replication *in vitro*. Microbiol Immunol 2003; 47(9): 681-4.
[http://dx.doi.org/10.1111/j.1348-0421.2003.tb03431.x] [PMID: 14584615]

[43] Chen H, Fu J, Chen H, *et al.* Ginger compound [6]-shogaol and its cysteine-conjugated metabolite (M2) activate Nrf2 in colon epithelial cells *in vitro* and *in vivo*. Chem Res Toxicol 2014; 27(9): 1575-85.
[http://dx.doi.org/10.1021/tx500211x] [PMID: 25148906]

[44] Yamamoto-Ribeiro MMG, Grespan R, Kohiyama CY, *et al.* Effect of *Zingiber officinale* essential oil on *Fusarium verticillioides* and fumonisin production. Food Chem 2013; 141(3): 3147-52. [http://dx.doi.org/10.1016/j.foodchem.2013.05.144] [PMID: 23871071]

[45] Ueno N, Hasebe T, Kaneko A, *et al.* TU-100 (Daikenchuto) and ginger ameliorate anti-CD3 antibody induced T cell-mediated murine enteritis: microbe-independent effects involving Akt and NF-κB suppression. PLoS One 2014; 9(5): e97456.
[http://dx.doi.org/10.1371/journal.pone.0097456] [PMID: 24857966]

[46] Alok A, Singh ID, Singh S, Kishore M, Jha PC. Curcumin – Pharmacological Actions And its Role in Oral Submucous Fibrosis: A Review. J Clin Diagn Res 2015; 9(10): ZE01-3. [http://dx.doi.org/10.7860/JCDR/2015/13857.6552] [PMID: 26557633]

[47] Ververidis F, Trantas E, Douglas C, Vollmer G, Kretzschmar G, Panopoulos N. Biotechnology of flavonoids and other phenylpropanoid-derived natural products. Part I: Chemical diversity, impacts on plant biology and human health. Biotechnol J 2007; 2(10): 1214-34. [http://dx.doi.org/10.1002/biot.200700084] [PMID: 17935117]

[48] Kaul TN, Middleton E Jr, Ogra PL. Antiviral effect of flavonoids on human viruses. J Med Virol 1985; 15(1): 71-9.
[http://dx.doi.org/10.1002/jmv.1890150110] [PMID: 2981979]

[49] Yi L, Li Z, Yuan K, *et al.* Small molecules blocking the entry of severe acute respiratory syndrome coronavirus into host cells. J Virol 2004; 78(20): 11334-9. [http://dx.doi.org/10.1128/JVI.78.20.11334-11339.2004] [PMID: 15452254]

[50] Villa TG, Feijoo-Siota L, Rama JLR, Ageitos JM. Antivirals against animal viruses. Biochem Pharmacol 2017; 133: 97-116.
[http://dx.doi.org/10.1016/j.bcp.2016.09.029] [PMID: 27697545]

[51] Ding S, Jiang H, Fang J. Regulation of immune function by polyphenols. J Immunol Res 2018; 2018: 1-8.

[http://dx.doi.org/10.1155/2018/1264074] [PMID: 29850614]

[52] Adem S, Eyupoglu V, Sarfraz I, Rasul A, Ali M. Identification of potent COVID-19 main protease (Mpro) inhibitors from natural polyphenols: an *in silico* strategy unveils a hope against CORONA. 2020.
[http://dx.doi.org/10.20944/preprints202003.0333.v1]

[53] Petr D, Marian H, David V, *et al.* Anti-inflammatory and antitumorpromoting effects of the triterpene acids from the leaves of Eriobotrya japonica. Nat Prod Rep 2006; 23: 394-411.

[54] Malinowska M, Sikora E, Ogonowski J. Production of triterpenoids with cell and tissue cultures. Acta Biochim Pol 2013; 60(4): 731-5.
[PMID: 24432325]

[55] Poehland BL, Carté BK, Francis TA, Hyland LJ, Allaudeen HS, Troupe N. *In vitro* antiviral activity of dammar resin triterpenoids. J Nat Prod 1987; 50(4): 706-13.
[http://dx.doi.org/10.1021/np50052a022] [PMID: 2828553]

[56] Cui J, Li F, Shi ZL. Origin and evolution of pathogenic coronaviruses. Nat Rev Microbiol 2019; 17(3): 181-92.
[http://dx.doi.org/10.1038/s41579-018-0118-9] [PMID: 30531947]

[57] St John SE, Tomar S, Stauffer SR, Mesecar AD. Targeting zoonotic viruses: Structure-based inhibition of the 3C-like protease from bat coronavirus HKU4--The likely reservoir host to the human coronavirus that causes Middle East Respiratory Syndrome (MERS). Bioorg Med Chem 2015; 23(17): 6036-48.
[http://dx.doi.org/10.1016/j.bmc.2015.06.039] [PMID: 26190463]

[58] Pandey R, Upadhayay P, Shukla SS. Plants having Anti-arthritic and Immunomodulator Potentials: An Review. Research Journal of Pharmacy and Technology 2017; 10(4): 1252-6.
[http://dx.doi.org/10.5958/0974-360X.2017.00222.0]

CHAPTER 6

Herbal Therapy for COVID-19

Upendra S. Bhadoriya[1,*], **Ankit Jain**[1] and **Sachin Kumar Jain**[1]

[1] *Oriental College of Pharmacy & Research Oriental University Ujjain Road Indore MP-452010, India*

Abstract: The Covid-19 epidemic is presently ravaging the world, claiming the lives of countless people. This health crisis is well recognised to be caused by SARS-CoV-2 infection, and the problem has yet to be remedied. Many modern doctors and researchers feel that a person's disease resistance ability is critical in battling viral infections. If used appropriately, herbal therapy can be a game changer in this case, since herbal drugs significantly boost or modify immune function, enhancing resistance to microbial infections. These drugs alter the cellular immune response, enhance immunity, impart antioxidant effect, raise IgG antibody production, activate macrophages, have anti-inflammatory and analgesic properties, and so relieve symptoms and reduce viral infection pathology development. Herbal medicine can also aid in the prevention of viral infections by blocking virus entrance and replication in the host cell. Due to their vast therapeutic capabilities, Curcumin, Shunthi, Bhumiamalki, Guduchi, Yashtimadhu, Pippali, and Haritaki, among other drugs, can be examined for their efficiency and safety against viral infection. The potential uses of herbal medicine as a supplementary and alternative treatment for SARS-CoV-2 illness were reviewed in this chapter. However, further research into the effects of herbal treatment in COVID-19 is needed.

Keywords: COVID-19, Health, Herbal therapy, Herbal therapy COVID-19, Immunity, Infection.

1. INTRODUCTION

As seen by the current situation, in which people all over the world are battling a new pandemic coronavirus disease, the history of human civilization has witnessed both wealthy advancement and different health calamities (COVID-19). The COVID-19 disease transmitted from humans to humans and was labeled a pandemic even after its initial period of occurrence. Due to its high rate of transmission and severity, COVID-19 is considered a current global health problem, with the medical community investing major efforts in combating it.

* **Corresponding author Upendra S. Bhadoriya:** IPS Academy College of Pharmacy, Rajendra Nagar AB Road, Indore MP-452012, India; E-mail: upendrabhadoriya@ipsacademy.org

This disorder is caused by the invasion of the zoonotic bacteria "severe acute respiratory syndrome coronavirus 2" (SARS-CoV-2) [1 - 3].

SARS-CoV-2 is an enveloped RNA virus that spreads by close contact and respiratory droplets when an infected person coughs or sneezes. The contaminated surface can also act as a source of transmission when a person contacts it before contacting his or her nose, mouth, or eyes [2 - 4].

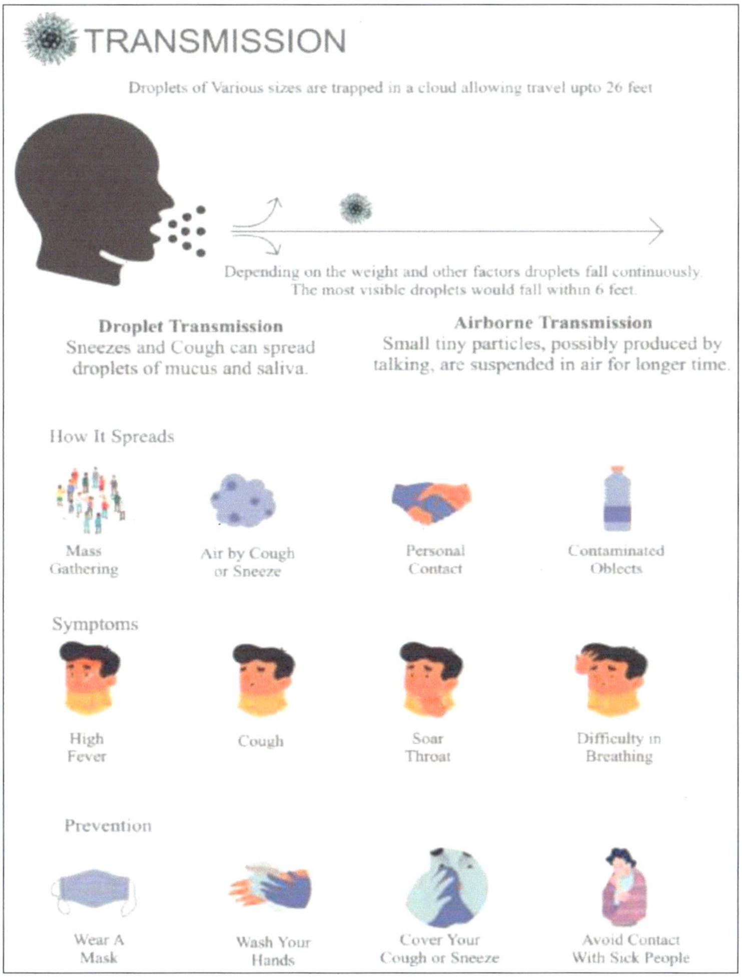

Fig. (1). Transmission, Symptoms and Prevention of COVID-19 Disease.

SARS-CoV-1 (2003), MERS-CoV (2012), and SARS-CoV-2 (2019) are three of the most common "respiratory syndrome coronaviruses" that are also lethal (4). SARS-CoV-2, which exhibits clinical symptoms comparable to those found in earlier respiratory syndrome coronaviruses, is connected to the current COVID-19 pandemic. The most frequent signs and symptoms are fever, cough, shortness of breath, and sore throat; however, muscular soreness and headache are also prevalent. Bilateral pneumonia, severe respiratory distress, and multi-organ failure, among others, are disease-related consequences that are important causes of death. Other signs of sickness include a loss of taste and smell, however, these only appear in the later stages of the disease [5, 6]. Fig. (**1**) depicts general considerations about COVID-19 disease propagation, symptoms, and prevention.

Frequent hand washing with soap, maintaining general and respiratory hygiene, avoiding frequent touching of the nose, eye, and face, disinfecting the floor or objects, wearing masks, avoiding close contact with the infected people, maintaining social distance, and using alcohol-based hand sanitizer are some of the preventive measures recommended by medical science. Pharmaceuticals such as favipiravir and Chloroquine, among others, are already used in conjunction with plasma treatment for illness management; however, vaccines are thought to have more favourable results, and scientists anticipate that the drugs will reach the experimental phase [1 - 4].

Researchers are presently concentrating their efforts on finding COVID-19 therapies, which include investigating the antiviral effects of botanicals and natural medications. Herbs have been reported to have antiviral effects against the SARS-CoV-2 virus [7]. Herbs are also thought to improve immunity, making them a vital part of the viral illness prevention strategy. However, it is important to establish the effectiveness and safety of herbal treatment against COVID-19 using experimental models. Herbs contain antiviral and immune-boosting qualities, thus they can help prevent SARS-CoV-2 illness from progressing and spreading. Herbal therapy can also be used as adjuvant and adjunct therapy in combination with standard COVID-19 therapies. Antiviral activity of plants or plant-based extracts has been found in trials against Coronavirus, Enterovirus, Dengue virus, Influenza virus, HIV, and Hepatitis B [1 - 3].

1.1. Herbal Therapy as a COVID-19 Treatment Option

Synthetic antivirals and immunomodulators failed to provide an appropriate therapeutic response against COVID-19, and emergency vaccination usage has yet to be licensed in certain countries, and even if it is, vaccine availability to the general public within a reasonable time period remains a challenge. As a result, alternative, supplemental, and adjuvant therapy techniques for COVID-19 infection prevention and treatment are needed. Fortunately, traditional medical practitioners established the efficiency of natural treatments even against severe viral illness, and herbal therapy may be useful in the treatment of COVID-19 (Fig.

2). Although further preclinical and clinical research is needed to establish the efficacy and safety of herbal therapy in certain situations, the fact that natural compounds may be useful to some extent is encouraging.

Herbal therapy can help fight the present pandemic in the following ways:

- Because many plants contain antiviral components, they can be used as an antiviral agent.
- Because many herbs help to increase immunity, herbal therapy can help to prevent infection.
- Herbs with essential oils can be utilised as an air disinfectant to prevent the spread of aerosols.
- Some natural substances have disinfection properties and can therefore be used as a surface sanitizer.

2. COVID-19 HERBAL THERAPY/HERBS

The creation of an effective and safe synthetic antiviral drug for COVID-19 therapy is a difficult task, and alterations in the viral genome impede medical researchers' efforts. Herbal therapy can be suggested as a safe, alternative, and complementary approach for the prevention and treatment of COVID-19 because there are no palliative or effective treatments available to combat this pandemic situation, and because the development and approval of vaccines are not moving at the rate that is required, and because the disease is still spreading.

2.1. *Echinacea Purpurea*

Because of its significant antiviral qualities, *Echinacea purpurea (E. purpurea)* is a popular herbal treatment used mostly in North America and Europe. Purple coneflower is a flower with extracts, teas, sprays, and tinctures available. Folkloric claims for respiratory ailments have been made in the United States [8, 9]. Chicoric acid, caffeic acids, polysaccharides, and alkylamides are some of the components that make it a useful medicinal plant [10]. It has been proved in several tests to be a useful antiviral medication for treating virus-related diseases. Echinacea extract is an antiviral medication, according to a research, since it has a direct virucidal action. Echinacea is thought to be particularly vulnerable to membrane-bound viruses; the MIC100 for herpes simplex and influenza viruses, respectively, was 0.39 g/mL and 0.58 g/mL. Because the human coronavirus is an enclosed virus, the MIC100 level has been found to be fairly high in non-membrane viruses; as a result, *E. purpurea* might be a potential therapeutic option for COVID-19 [11]. Furthermore, some Echinacea preparations claim to have immunomodulatory and immunostimulatory properties; research indicated that it enhances the production of various cytokines that support immune cell function. Because Echinacea possesses both virucidal and immunostimulatory capabilities, its effectiveness against COVD19, as well as its safety profile, may be investigated.

2.2. Curcumin

The rhizomatous herbal plant turmeric is known scientifically as *Curcuma longa (C. longa)* (Fig. **3h**). *Curcuma longa* is a plant with several medicinal characteristics, thus researchers have been working hard to find new applications for it. For millennia, it has been used as a spice, natural food colourant, and flavouring ingredient. Antioxidant, anti-inflammatory, anticancer, anti-diabetic, and neuroprotective activities have been shown in *C. longa* [12, 13]. Curcumin is composed of carbohydrates, proteins, lipids, minerals, curcuminoids, demethoxycurcumin, and bisdemethoxycurcumin, all of which have a role in the therapeutic activities of curcumin.

Curcumin helps to treat hypertension by blocking angiotensin II receptor type-1, which lowers blood pressure. Blood artery constriction, a decrease in renal and other tissues' perfusion, and a fall in blood pressure are all prevented by this procedure [14]. One of COVID-19's most prevalent comorbidities is hypertension, which occurs when the level of angiotensin-converting enzyme increases [15]. Antihypertensive medicines that inhibit the angiotensin-converting enzyme can thus be used to reduce the risk of hypertension caused by SARS-CoV-2 infection.

Curcumin also suppresses proinflammatory cytokines, making it anti-inflammatory [16]. Curcumin also boosts the immune system's production of IL-6 and TNF- [17]. Curcumin's use as a COVID-19 supplemental or alternative medicine is called into question by these findings. More study is needed, however, to verify curcumin's efficacy in the treatment and prevention of COVID-19.

2.3. *Cinchona SP.,*

The cinchona tree, *Chincona* L. in technical terms, is a valuable medicinal herb, especially in the case of fever (Fig. **3o**) [18]. Quinine alkaloids, which are present in tree bark, are used to cure malaria. It is generally known that quinine sulphate was regarded to be the most effective therapy for COVID-19 at the start of the present pandemic. Chloroquine and hydroxychloroquine have antiviral activity against SARS-CoV infection, according to a research study [19], hence quinine, a chloroquine analogue, might be helpful for COVID-19 patients. Because cinchona includes quinine, it must be backed up by acceptable safety evidence in COVID-19 cases. Quinine's antiviral impact is connected to protein heat shock response activation, interfering with virus replication pathways, and NF-kB regulation by blocking. Cinchona's primary alkaloid Quinine has both immunostimulant and immunosuppressive effects against viral infections; it increases the synthesis of the cytokine IFN-, therefore it can be used as an immunostimulant to prevent virus invasion. As a result, it is possible that cinchona bark extract will help with COVID-19 disease [20, 21].

2.4. *Withania Somnifera*

It is a little shrub with pale green blooms, simple leaves, and crimson-colored berries. Ashwagandha is another name for Indian ginseng (Fig. **3n**). The majority of the benefits come from Ashwagandha's root and leaves. The leaves are most commonly used to make tea. The root may be eaten in a variety of ways, but it is most commonly dried, powdered, and taken as a supplement these days. Blood sugar levels, cortisol levels, depressive symptoms, and inflammation can all be reduced with ashwagandha extract. It promotes the enhanced strength, muscle mass, and cerebral ability. Ashwagandha improves the body's resilience to illness by enhancing cell-mediated immunity. It also contains strong antioxidant properties that aid in the protection of cells from free radical damage. It also demonstrated inhibitory capabilities against a variety of malignancies (breast, colon, prostate, colon, ovarian, lung, and brain), as well as the mechanisms and pathways involved [22 - 25]. Ashwagandha extracts have been found to have a significant impact on immunological health and stress reduction [25].

2.5. *Planax Quinquefolius* (Ginseng)

Ginseng is a plant of the Araliaceae family and the genus Panax, with the formal name Panax ginseng C. A. Meyer and the title of "King of Herbs" in traditional herbal medicine (Fig. **3k**) [26]. COVID-19-induced acute respiratory tract infection, influenza, or chronic disorders pose a serious hazard to human health around the world. Ginseng can boost human immunity against acute respiratory tract infection due to its Qi-beneficial action [27].

2.6. Fenugreek

Is there a well-known Ayurvedic herb that serves as a natural anti-oxidant and boosts the immune system? It's used as herb (dry or fresh leaves), spice (seeds), and vegetable (fresh leaves), as well as a condiment in artificial maple syrup flavour and steroid manufacturing [28].

2.7. Herbal Extracts and Nutraceuticals [29]

2.7.1. Vitamins

Obese people, healthcare workers, and smokers should take 20-50 g of vitamin D per day to boost their resistance to COVID-19 infection, according to new research.

2.7.2. Minerals in the Diet

Selenium

The significance of selenium in immunological function.

Zinc

Zinc deficiency is common among the elderly, which is necessary for immunological function.

Iron

The tight management of serum iron concentration may thus result in better clinical results for COVID-19 patients.

N-acetyl-cysteine Amino Acid (NAC)

NAC, which is produced from the naturally occurring amino acid cysteine, is most typically administered to people who have respiratory problems.

2.7.3. Probiotics

Probiotic nutritional supplementation has been shown to be useful for people with respiratory tract infections.

2.7.4. Omega-3 fatty Acids

Omega-3 fatty acids have been shown to be beneficial in lowering airway inflammation and bronchoconstriction, as well as in fighting viral infections, therefore its application against COVID-19 bears further research.

2.8. *Tinospora Cordifolia* (Giloy, Guduchi)

Giloy or Guduchi, scientific name *Tinospora cordifolia*, is a plant that has been utilised for medical purposes for millennia (Fig. **3d**). Giloy's hypolipidemic, hypoglycemic, hepatoprotective, antibacterial, anti-inflammatory, antiosteoporotic, antiobesity, anticarcinogenic, and antimutagenic activities have been found in numerous investigations [17]. Various diterpene compounds and polysaccharides, notably arabinogalactan polysaccharide, are thought to be present in Guduchi or Giloy plant. Immunomodulating and adaptogenic polysaccharides and terpenoids are found in nature. Several investigations on Giloy herbal extract have shown that it can generate significant increases in IgG antibodies in the blood, macrophage activation, cell regulated immunity, and humoral immunity [18].

2.9. *Ocimum Sanctum,* (Holy Basil, Tulsi)

Tulsi is a type of basil that is also known as holy basil (Fig. **3e**). Many *in-vitro* and *in-vivo* studies on animals and humans have demonstrated its therapeutic potential as an antioxidant, anti-aging, anticancer, and antiviral agent. It also has antimicrobial properties, immunomodulatory activity, immunomodulatory activity, antipyretic activity, and anti-arthritic activity, and potential for treatment of gum ulcers, kidney problems, earache, menstrual irregularities, arthritis, anorexia, and malaria, and as a haemoglobin replacement therapy. Tulsi's role in providing scientific data against COVID-19 has also been clarified.

2.10. *Syzygium Aromaticum* (Clove, Laung)

Syzygium aromaticum is the scientific name for clove (Fig. **3i**). Consuming whole cloves is an excellent way to enhance your immune system. Clove essential oil may have nutritional therapeutic potential due to its diverse effects, which include antimicrobial, antifungal, antiviral, anti-inflammatory, cytotoxic, analgesic, and anaesthetic activities, as well as being very potent antioxidants and inhibiting the post-binding entry of the SARS coronavirus into cells. Anti-platelet actions, on the other hand, prevent the formation of a thrombus or blood clot. As a result, clove essential oil may be one of the best possibilities for combating the Coronavirus and protecting against sudden death seen in some Corona virus-infected patients due to embolism and hypercoagulable development. Clove Oil should only be diffused in well-ventilated areas, and treatment sessions should not last longer than 60 minutes [21].

2.11. *Sambucus Nigra* (Elderberry)

Elderberry, scientifically known as *Sambucus nigra*, is a deep purple berry found throughout Europe and Western Asia (Fig. **3a**). It's been in use for a long time because of its numerous health benefits. It contains polyphenolic compounds (Anthocyanins, Flavonols, Phenolic acid), terpenes, carbohydrates (mostly glucose and fructose), citric acid, malic acid, lectins, and other necessary nutrients [2]. *In vitro*, liquid elderberry extract has antiviral properties against influenza and respiratory bacterial infections. Elderberry (*Sambucus nigra* L. (Adoxaceae)) has been shown in preclinical studies to suppress the replication and viral attachment of the human Corona virus NL63 (HCoV-NL63), which is related to COVID-19 and belongs to the corona virus family. Elderberry is the most effective early-stage prevention or treatment for corona virus infections [8]. Their nutrient contents per 100 grams, on the other hand, include 870 mg Vitamin A, 34.10 mg Vitamin C, 391.33 mg Potassium, 28.06 mg Calcium, 1.86 mg Iron, 217 mg Sodium, as well as several other minerals, folic acid, amino acids, and dietary fibres. This fruit is high in flavonoids, which have antioxidant and anti-inflammatory characteristics and help preserve healthy cells from damaging free radicals, which has implications in skin care and boosting immunity.

2.12. *Allium Sativum* (Garlic, Lahsun)

Garlic is abundant in antioxidants and aids in the reduction of stress and high blood pressure (Fig. **3b**). It also aids in the absorption of thiamine (vitamin B1) in the body and prevents beriberi. Colds, flu, and COVID-19 infection may be less severe as a result of the antiviral property. Garlic, as a result, strengthens the immune system and aids in the battle against viruses and other disorders. It contains Allicin, a broad-spectrum antibiotic [11]. It has been suggested that it improves immunological health by boosting the protection of white blood cells such as NK cells and macrophages [12]. In an *in vitro* study13, *Allium sativum* L. (Amaryllidaceae) extract suppressed the synthesis of viral nucleoproteins and polymerase activity, suppressing influenza A (H1N1) virus. For colds, the study suggested an *Allium cepa* L. (Amaryllidaceae) decoction [8, 14]. Garlic should always be chopped or crushed before eating since it gives more nutrients when exposed to oxygen. Garlic is used to flavour nearly every type of food on the planet [2].

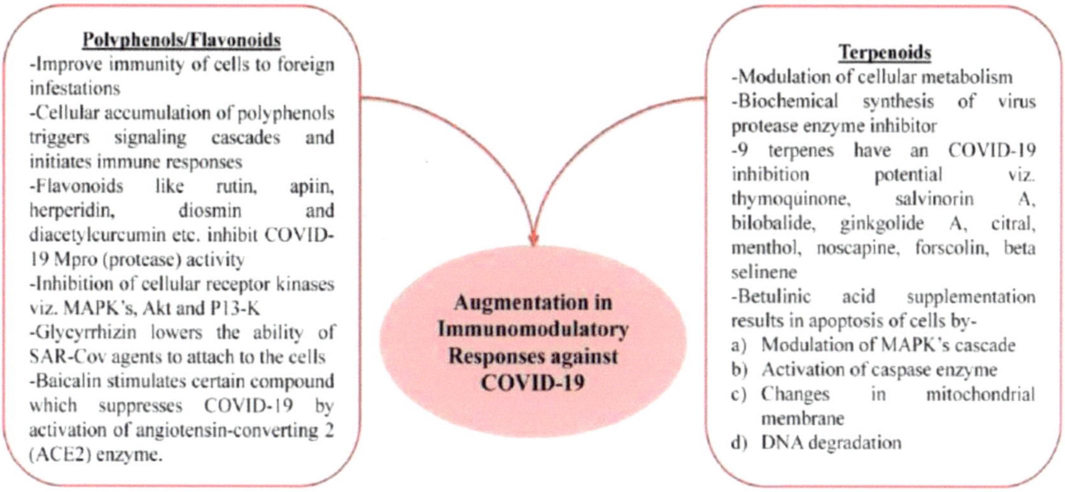

Fig. (2). Prospects of Augmentation in Immuno-Modulatory Responses against COVID-19 by Polyphenols/Flavonoids and Terpenoids.

2.13. *Zingiber Officinalis* (Ginger)

Zingiber officinale Roscoe is another name for Zanjabeel or Adrak (Fig. **3c**). It is a very important medicinal plant that belongs to the Zingiberaceae family, among other things. Ginger's anti-inflammatory, antifungal, and anti-cancer effects are well-known. Ginger has long been used to treat colds and coughs, nausea, asthma, travel sickness, morning sickness, arthritis, gastrointestinal issues, and even depression in traditional medicine. People use it to make ginger tea by crushing ginger and boiling it with tea leaves and water. Since ancient times, powdered ginger combined with pulverised cloves, cardamom, and caraway has been used to treat digestive problems. It is immunosuppressive (boosts up the immune system of the patients which further prevents the load of infection). 15 Ginger is useful in the treatment of respiratory disorders (relieves congestion associated with the common cold).

2.14. Traditional Indian Medicines

In India, the AYUSH ministry has given special attention to the use of natural resources to manage pandemic diseases. In this case, it was indicated that the use of a natural ayurvedic formulation like Chyavanprash to boost immunity against viral infection could be beneficial. Home remedies such as milk with turmeric powder, Tulsi decoction, cinnamon, and black pepper have also been advised. Guduchi, Shunthi, Bhumiamalki, Yashtimadhu, Haritaki, Pippali, and Maricha are natural herbs that may be effective in preventing viral infection by modifying the immunological response.

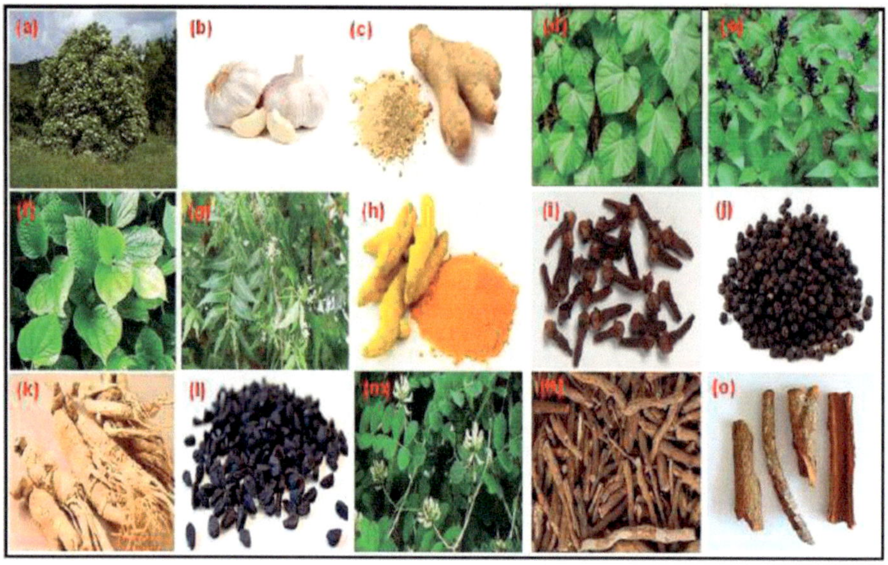

Fig. (3). Different plants and herbs that can help in the fight against COVID-19. (a) Elderberry, *Sambucuss nigra* (b) Garlic, *Allium sativum* (c) Ginger, *Zingiber officinalis* (d) Giloy, *Tinospora cordifolia* (e) Tulsi, *Ocimum sanctum* (f) Betalvive, *Piper betal* (g) Margosa, *Azadirachtin indica* (h) Turmeric, *Curuma domestica* (i) Clove, *Syzgium aromaticum* (j) Black paper, *Piper nigrum* (k) Ginseng, *Planax quinquefolius* (l) Black cumin, *Black cumin L.* (m) Licorice astragalus, *Astragalus glycyphyllos* (n) Aswagandha, *Withania Somnifera* (o) Cinchona (*Cinchona officinalis*).

Guduchi (*Tinospora cardifolia*) is a popular plant known for its immunomodulatory and antioxidant effects. Guduchi is thought to promote immunological response; it primarily affects humoral and cell-mediated immunity, increases IgG antibody production, and stimulates macrophages to fight viral infection. As a result, its utility in COVID-19 infection must be determined in order to discover natural alternatives to the current pandemic outbreak.

Bhumiamalki (*Phyllanphus niruri*) is an antiviral, hepatoprotective, hypoglycaemic, antibacterial, anti-inflammatory, and analgesic shrub. Bhumiamalki has antiviral and antioxidant activities due to the presence of constituents such as phenols, tannins, and flavonoids. The antimicrobial properties of *Phyllanphus niruri* are related to specific components such as glucosides, gallocatechin, and rutin.

Shunthi (*Zingiber officinale*) is a spice with alkaloids, volatile oils, vitamins, minerals, and phenol. Many therapeutic benefits of herbs, such as antibacterial, analgesic, and antiulcer qualities, are attributed to these components. Shunthi has antiviral properties as well as improving immunological response. Its antioxidant activity may potentially provide health advantages in viral infection-induced oxidative damage to biological constituents.

Yashtimadhu (*Glycyrrhiza glabra*) is a medicinal plant whose root (Fig. **3m**), in particular, contains phenolic chemicals that aid in the treatment of respiratory tract infections. Its principal ingredients, such as triterpene, saponins, and glycyrrhizin acid, among others, have antibacterial properties and are helpful in viral infections, particularly those involving the respiratory system.

Haritaki (*Terminalia chebula*) is a medicinal plant high in Gallic acid and tannins which give it antiviral properties. It also has anti-inflammatory and antipyretic properties, making it useful for viral infection-induced inflammatory symptoms (Fig. **3j**).

Maricha (*Piper nigrum*) is another natural herb with a wide range of medicinal effects, which could be attributable to the presence of ingredients such as serine, carotene, and ascorbic acid, among others. It has anti-inflammatory, anti-oxidant, anti-microbial, and antipyretic properties, making it effective for viral infections in diabetes patients who are prone to inflammatory cold and cough symptoms.

Pippali (*Piper longum*) is a natural chemical that contains lignans, alkaloids, and esters (Fig. **3l**). It has antiviral properties and is used to treat respiratory infections. Piperine, the key ingredient responsible for the plant's medicinal properties, also relieves inflammatory symptoms associated with fever and infection.

All of the herbs or plants mentioned above have a therapeutic value for preventing and treating a viral infection in the current pandemic condition. These plants' antiviral properties may be useful for reducing viral load. Furthermore, the antipyretic activity of natural remedies aids in the reduction of increased temperature in cases of fever caused by a viral illness. Furthermore, anti-inflammatory plants inhibit inflammatory symptoms of illness by calming inflammatory mediators. It is also clear that COVID-19 is exacerbated by diabetes and hypertension, thus natural therapies with anti-diabetic and anti-hypertensive properties may provide additional health benefits in addition to preventing COVID-19 disease's devastating implications. Natural medications that can change or enhance immune responses could be used as a preventive therapy to limit SARS-CoV-2 infection and pathology progression [19]. Traditional herbs/plants such as Curcumin, Guduchi, Shunthi, Bhumiamalki, Yashtimadhu, Haritaki, Pippali, and Maricha, among others, need to be examined further for their efficacy and safety against COVID-19 infection, according to literature data.

2.15. Rebooting of the Immune System

The enhancement of the body's immunological reactions is the cutting edge in fending off diseases and remaining healthy. To do this, it is necessary to change one's existing lifestyle by adding smarter tasks to one's to-do list in order to make one's internal immune/defense system competitive against viruses like COVID-19. This would naturally cure the antiviral effects within the body by removing the disease's and infection's avidity. The majority of these characteristics are tied to reactivating anti-inflammatory functions, improving cell-mediated immune functions, modulating APC (Antigen Presenting Cell) activities, and reducing pro-inflammatory mediators, all of which are linked to better immunity. They also play a role in successful cell-to-cell communication during both innate and adaptive immune responses [23].

As a result, a scientific expedition aimed at boosting the immune system through proper sleep, judicious exercise, a stress-free environment, proper nutritive foods, adequate water intake, and consumption of fresh and healthy fruits and vegetables would expect citizens to cope with coronavirus outbreaks by naturally vaccinating their systems [24]. Different stressors, lack of sleep, and carbonated beverages are thought to suppress the immune system by releasing ACTH (Adrenocorticotrophic Hormones), which include adrenaline, non-adrenaline, and glucocorticoids. As a result, a person's immune system is weakened, making them more susceptible to harmful illnesses. Immune system mediators such as NK (Natural Killer) cells, Helper-T-cells, lymphocytes, antibodies, interleukins (IL4, 5, 10, 13), and cytokines, for example, are weakened, leading to an increased risk of infection and the reactivation of latent viruses [25]. Furthermore, lack of sleep may impair an individual's immunological pathways through ACTH-stimulated prolonged activation of NF-B, which increases the risk of infection due to decreased microbial gene expression levels. Meanwhile, enough sleep regulates the body's hormonal responses, allowing T-cells to reorganise towards lymph nodes and boost their immunogenic memory response [26]. Furthermore, drinking carbonated beverages or alcoholic beverages induces high blood glucose or CO_2, which leads to hypercapnia, which inhibits macrophage function and pathogen clearance. Immuno-modulators are also hampered, resulting in a lack of control over invading pathogens. Proper sleep, an active daily routine, exercise, and other factors boost immune surveillance in the form of NK cells, monocytes, neutrophils, T-cells, Immunoglobulin, and other factors to combat negative health effects [27]. Apart from that, the intake of multivitamins within the human body can help to wash away disease forces by recruiting immune warriors [28]. Multivitamin-rich diets have immuno-modulatory properties on a variety of immune cells, including monocytes, neutrophils, lymphocytes, NK cells, and dendritic cells, which boost immunity against infections [29]. Exacerbating the levels of Cathelicidin, Defensin, antimicrobial peptides, phagocytosis, neutrophil migration and chemotaxis, oxidant generation, NK-activation (CD69, CD25), IF-, antibodies synthesis, cytokine synthesis, and T-cell proliferation, these immune cells may trigger anti-pathogenic responses against coronaviruses [30].

2.16. COVID-19 Herbal Therapy: The Role of Specific Phyto-constituents

Different phyto-elements, such as tannins, alkaloids, saponins, glycosides, polyphenol, and other biologically important constituents, can be found in many parts of the plant, including seeds, leaves, bark, fruits, and roots. These plant constituents all have a variety of pharmacological properties, including antiviral activity. This section discussed the antiviral properties of various plant elements and how they might work against viral infection [18].

The following Method is Used by These Plant Ingredients to Prevent Viral Infections:

- Restriction of viral entrance and replication inhibits viral infection.
- Change viral envelope glycoproteins to prevent viral infection.
- The production of nucleocapsid protein, which is required for viral replication, is reduced by several phytoconstituents.
- At an early stage of infection, several phyto-constituents impede the virus's absorption and penetration.
- Interferes with the encoding of genes, resulting in antiviral action.
- The majority of plant constituents have the ability to boost immunological responses to microbial diseases.
- By limiting virus shedding and budding at the cell membrane, you can avoid retroviral infection.
- Another way by which some plant elements protect against viral infection is by inhibiting translation initiation.
- Some phyto-constituents block proteases and hinder the phosphorylation process.

As shown in Table **1**, there are various targeted components detected in the COVID virus for drug candidates. By targeting these elements, drug candidates can exert anti-SARS-CoV-2 activity.

Table 1. Possible drug target for anti-SARS-CoV-2 activity of natural medicines.

S. No.	Herbal Drugs	Possible Drug Target For Covid-19
1	*Tribulus terrestris*	Papain-like protease [31]

(Table 1) cont.....

S. No.	Herbal Drugs	Possible Drug Target For Covid-19
2	*Ocimum sanctum*	Papain-like protease [32]
3	*Withania Somnifera*	3C-like main protease [33]
4	*Curcuma longa*	3C-like main protease [34]
5	*Phyllanthus emblica*	Spike and Helicase protein [35]
6	*Allium cepa*	SARS-CoV NTPase/helicase [36]
7	*Zingiber officinale*	SARS-CoV 3a protein [37]
8	*Galla chinensis*	SARS-CoV S protein-ACE2 [38]
9	*Cannabis sativa*	Protein pre-requisite for SARS-CoV2 invasion into host cells [39]
10	*Glycyrrhiza glabra*	Counter balance the activeness of COVID-19 and could be used as an antiviral drug [40]
11	*Porphyridium* sp.	Corona Viruses that inhibit the binding or internalization of virus into the host cells [41]
12	*Nilavembu Kudineer*	Immuno-modulatory activity against ACE2 enzyme receptor, that routes virus entry in the pathogenesis of Novel Coronavirus [42]
13	*Camellia sinensis*	Target COVID-19 main protease (Mpro), key enzyme of Coronavirus involved in virus replication and transcription [43]
14	*Lawsonia inermis*	Phytochemical, cytotoxicity and anti-inflammatory actions confirmed in fractions of extract as observed as a potent constituents [44]
15	*Ginkgo biloba*	Impeded DNA and protein synthesis by binding towards host cell receptors to activate cell-signaling pathways [45]
16	*Silybum marianum, Withania Somnifera*, Tinospora cordiofolia and *Aloe barbadensis*	Spike (S) glycoproteins, main protease (Mpro) and RNAdependent RNA-polymerases (RdRp) [46]
17	*Betula pubescens*	Inhibitory compounds against MERS-CoV 3C-like proteases (3CLpro) [47]
18	*Exocarpium Citri grandis*	Antitussive, expectorant, improved lung function, pulmonary fibrosis, and antiviral immune response [48]
19	*Alpinia officinarum*	SARS-CoV-2 papain-like protease (PLpro) inhibitors [49]

2.16.1. Phenolic Compounds

Tannins, particularly phlorofucofuroeckol and dieckol, are well-known for their capacity to prevent viral infection by limiting viral entry and reproduction. Pomegranate polyphenols have the ability to alter viral envelope glycoproteins.

Procyanidins, for example, prevent viral infection by interfering with the reproduction process. Some polyphenols stop viruses from infecting people by rendering them non-infectious, resulting in compromised envelopes. It was previously recognised that resveratrol (polyphenol) inhibits MERS-CoV respiratory infection and enhances cellular survival after viral infection by lowering the expression of nucleocapsid protein, which is necessary for viral replication. MERS is a respiratory viral infection caused by the corona virus, which has a clinical spectrum similar to SARS-CoV-2, which causes COVID-19. As a result, polyphenols that are active against MERS-CoV respiratory infection can be examined to see if they are also active against SARS-CoV-2 [50].

2.16.2. Saponins

Saponins, such as saikosaponins, found in medicinal plants such as Bupleurum spp. and Heteromorpha spp., have biological properties such as antiviral activity. Saikosaponin-B2 is an anti-coronaviral saponin whose mode of action is thought to be interference in the early stages of viral replication, including virus absorption and penetration. Similarly, oleanane triterpenes have antiviral properties, preventing viral replication and interfering with gene expression. Similarly, Escin derivatives derived from Aesculus turbinata seed have inhibitory effects on viral propagation. Bioactive components from *Nigella sativa*, such as nigellimine, have structural similarities to Chloroquine and hydro-xychloroquine, so it's possible that this substance can stimulate immune response during viral infection [51].

2.16.3. Alkaloids

Lycorine, an alkaloid mostly obtained from Amaryllidaceae species, has anti-viral activity against SARS-CoV. Alkaloids are natural compounds produced from plant sources that have a variety of biological functions, including anti-viral properties. Tylophorine compounds are *in-vitro* inhibitors of enteropathogenic coronaviruses; a study found that tylophorine compounds (EC50 values 5-340 nM) significantly reduced the cytopathic effect generated by SARS CoV during an *in-vitro* assay [52].

2.16.4. Polysaccharides

Polysaccharides, a common natural component present in many plants, have a wide range of biological actions, including antiviral activity. *In vitro*, Astragalus polysaccharides suppressed the replication of the virus that causes infectious bronchitis, which was related to lower mRNA levels of the inflammatory cytokines IL-6, IL-8, IL-1B, and TNF-. Similarly, Ginkgo biloba polysaccharides block virus attachment and entrance into cells, resulting in antiviral benefits against a variety of viral illnesses [53].

2.16.5. Anthraquinones

Anthraquinones, which are derived from a variety of plant species, are known for their distinctive pharmacological reactions, including strong antimicrobial activity. Because they have the ability to suppress virus shedding and budding at the cell membrane, pseudohypericin and hypericin can impede retroviral infection. It was also thought that anthraquinones' antiviral effect was linked to the inhibition of protein kinase phosphorylation when cells were infected with retroviruses. Some natural drugs in this class are powerful translation initiation inhibitors and SARS-CoV protease inhibitors [54].

3. HERBAL THERAPY'S FUTURE PROSPECTS AGAINST COVID-19 AND OVERCOMING CHALLENGES

Herbal medicines have been used for a variety of health benefits for many years, and natural medicines were once thought to be life-saving therapies due to their safe biological profile. Herbal therapy produces a therapeutic response with no serious side effects; however, their pharmacokinetic profile must be researched and optimized in order to overcome the problems of poor abortion and low bioavailability. As a result, modern dosage forms are necessary for the administration of herbal medications [55].

The advantages of using innovative carriers to carry medicines include the capacity to distribute drugs at the desired rate while also delivering active constituents to the site of action, improving bioavailability. In the case of viral infection, nanoparticles, liposomes, nanocapsules, nanoemulsion, and phytosomes, among others, can be utilised to deliver herbal medicines as part of herbal therapy. When these drug carriers are used in herbal therapy, the undesired toxicity of the herbal medicine can be hidden. Herbal medicines' solubility, stability, specificity, and selectivity can all be improved with a new drug delivery method. As a result, innovative drug delivery systems or nano-carriers can be employed to overcome pharmacokinetic issues associated with herbal therapy, particularly in disorders like COVID-19, where fast and prolonged therapeutic activity is essential [56].

However, there are a number of issues with herbal medication therapy that must be addressed when it is advised for pandemic outbreaks. These issues include the following:

1. There is a need for preclinical and clinical research data on herbal therapy's effectiveness against SARS-CoV-2.

2. Standardization of herbal medications is required to ensure their quality and quantity.

3. Toxicological testing to ensure the safety of herbal medicines when used long-term in COVID-19 patients.

4. Regulatory control for the use of herbal medications must be established using a proven quality control and standardization system.

5. To expand the global usefulness of herbal medicine, it is necessary to raise awareness and public belief in its ability to handle pandemic situations.

FINAL THOUGHTS/CONCLUSION

Herbal medicine can be created as a complementary and alternative therapy to the COVID-19 validated therapy. By modifying cellular and humoral immune responses, these medications can assist to avoid infection. Herbal therapy can assist in enhancing immunity against SARS-CoV-2 infection by interfering with viral invasion and replication. However, experimental investigations on the effects of herbal therapy in COVID-19 are required. Aside from using treatment measures such as synthetic or herbal pharmaceuticals, it is also recommended to employ preventive measures such as using an air-disinfectant, a surface sanitizing agent, maintaining social distance, and wearing a face mask, among other things.

CONSENT FOR PUBLICATION

Not applicable.

CONFLICT OF INTEREST

The author declares no conflict of interest, financial or otherwise.

ACKNOWLEDGEMENTS

Declared none.

REFERENCES

[1] Wang C, Horby PW, Hayden FG, Gao GF. A novel coronavirus outbreak of global health concern. Lancet 2020; 395(10223): 470-3.
[http://dx.doi.org/10.1016/S0140-6736(20)30185-9] [PMID: 31986257]

[2] Bedford J, Enria D, Giesecke J, *et al.* COVID-19: towards controlling of a pandemic. Lancet 2020; 395(10229): 1015-8.
[http://dx.doi.org/10.1016/S0140-6736(20)30673-5] [PMID: 32197103]

[3] Di Gennaro F, Pizzol D, Marotta C, *et al.* Coronavirus diseases (COVID-19) current status and future perspectives: a narrative review. Int J Environ Res Public Health 2020; 17(8): 2690.
[http://dx.doi.org/10.3390/ijerph17082690] [PMID: 32295188]

[4] Chen N, Zhou M, Dong X, *et al.* Epidemiological and clinical characteristics of 99 cases of 2019 novel coronavirus pneumonia in Wuhan, China: a descriptive study. Lancet 2020; 395(10223): 507-13.
[http://dx.doi.org/10.1016/S0140-6736(20)30211-7] [PMID: 32007143]

[5] Menni C, Valdes A, Freydin MB. Loss of smell and taste in combination with other symptoms is a strong predictor of COVID-19 infection. MedRxiv 2020.
[http://dx.doi.org/10.1101/2020.04.05.20048421]

[6] Yang Y, Islam MS, Wang J, Li Y, Chen X. Traditional Chinese medicine in the treatment of patients infected with 2019-New Coronavirus (SARS-CoV-2): a review and perspective. Int J Biol Sci 2020; 16(10): 1708-17.
[http://dx.doi.org/10.7150/ijbs.45538] [PMID: 32226288]

[7] Sharma M, Anderson SA, Schoop R, Hudson JB. Induction of multiple pro-inflammatory cytokines by respiratory viruses and reversal by standardized Echinacea, a potent antiviral herbal extract. Antiviral Res 2009; 83(2): 165-70.
[http://dx.doi.org/10.1016/j.antiviral.2009.04.009] [PMID: 19409931]

[8] Hudson J, Vimalanathan S. Echinacea-a source of potent antivirals for respiratory virus infections. Pharmaceuticals (Basel) 2011; 4(7): 1019-31.
[http://dx.doi.org/10.3390/ph4071019]

[9] Barnes J, Anderson LA, Gibbons S, Phillipson JD. *Echinacea* species (*Echinacea angustifolia* (DC.) Hell., *Echinacea pallida* (Nutt.) Nutt., *Echinacea purpurea* (L.) Moench): a review of their chemistry, pharmacology and clinical properties. J Pharm Pharmacol 2010; 57(8): 929-54.
[http://dx.doi.org/10.1211/0022357056127] [PMID: 16102249]

[10] Burger RA, Torres AR, Warren RP, Caldwell VD, Hughes BG. Echinacea-induced cytokine production by human macrophages. Int J Immunopharmacol 1997; 19(7): 371-9.
[http://dx.doi.org/10.1016/S0192-0561(97)00061-1] [PMID: 9568541]

[11] Huang C, Wang Y, Li X, *et al.* Clinical features of patients infected with 2019 novel coronavirus in Wuhan, China. Lancet 2020; 395(10223): 497-506.
[http://dx.doi.org/10.1016/S0140-6736(20)30183-5] [PMID: 31986264]

[12] Hadi A, Pourmasoumi M, Ghaedi E, Sahebkar A. The effect of Curcumin/Turmeric on blood pressure modulation: A systematic review and meta-analysis. Pharmacol Res 2019; 150: 104505.
[http://dx.doi.org/10.1016/j.phrs.2019.104505] [PMID: 31647981]

[13] Lekshmi PC, Arimboor R, Nisha VM, Menon AN, Raghu KG. *In vitro* antidiabetic and inhibitory potential of turmeric *(Curcuma longa* L) rhizome against cellular and LDL oxidation and angiotensin converting enzyme. J Food Sci Technol 2014; 51(12): 3910-7.
[http://dx.doi.org/10.1007/s13197-013-0953-7] [PMID: 25477660]

[14] Alhenc-Gelas F, Bouby N, Girolami JP. Kallikrein/K1, kinins, and ACE/kininase II in homeostasis and in disease insight from human and experimental genetic studies, therapeutic implication. Front Med (Lausanne) 2019; 6: 136.
[http://dx.doi.org/10.3389/fmed.2019.00136] [PMID: 31316987]

[15] Zisman LS. ACE and ACE2: a tale of two enzymes. Eur Heart J 2005; 26(4): 322-4. [http://dx.doi.org/10.1093/eurheartj/ehi043] [PMID: 15671047]

[16] Leong XF. The spice for hypertension: protective role of Curcuma longa. Biomed Pharmacol J 2018; 11(4): 1829-40. [http://dx.doi.org/10.13005/bpj/1555]

[17] Fang L, Karakiulakis G, Roth M. Are patients with hypertension and diabetes mellitus at increased risk for COVID-19 infection? Lancet Respir Med 2020; 8(4): e21. [http://dx.doi.org/10.1016/S2213-2600(20)30116-8] [PMID: 32171062]

[18] Coronavirus Disease 2019 (COVID-19) – Symptoms. 2020.

[19] Prasansuklab A, Theerasri A, Rangsinth P, Sillapachaiyaporn C, Chuchawankul S, Tencomnao T. Anti-COVID-19 drug candidates: A review on potential biological activities of natural products in the management of new coronavirus infection. J Tradit Complement Med 2021; 11(2): 144-57. [http://dx.doi.org/10.1016/j.jtcme.2020.12.001] [PMID: 33520683]

[20] Arshad MS, Khan U, Sadiq A, *et al.* Coronavirus disease (COVID-19) and immunity booster green foods: A mini review. Food Sci Nutr 2020; 8(8): 3971-6. [http://dx.doi.org/10.1002/fsn3.1719] [PMID: 32837716]

[21] Srivastava AK, Chaurasia JP, Khan R, Dhand C, Verma S. Role of Medicinal plants of Traditional Use in Recuperating Devastating COVID-19 Situation. Med Aromat Plants (Los Angeles) 2020; 9: 359.

[22] https://www.merriam-webster.com/dictionary/immunity

[23] Robin R, Fiona R, Elaine M. "Pathology Illustrated- Immunity", 7th Edition, 2011; 87-111.

[24] Akira S, Uematsu S, Takeuchi O. Pathogen recognition and innate immunity. Cell 2006; 124(4): 783-801. [http://dx.doi.org/10.1016/j.cell.2006.02.015] [PMID: 16497588]

[25] Babich O, Sukhikh S, Prosekov A, Asyakina L, Ivanova S. Medicinal Plants to Strengthen Immunity during a Pandemic. Pharmaceuticals (Basel) 2020; 13(10): 313. [http://dx.doi.org/10.3390/ph13100313] [PMID: 33076514]

[26] Vulic J, Vracar L, Sumic Z. Chemical characteristics of cultivated elderberry fruit. Acta Period Technol 2008; 39(39): 85-90. [http://dx.doi.org/10.2298/APT0839085V]

[27] Torabian G, Valtchev P, Adil Q, Dehghani F. Anti-influenza activity of elderberry (Sambucus nigra). J Funct Foods 2019; 54: 353-60. [http://dx.doi.org/10.1016/j.jff.2019.01.031]

[28] Schoeman D, Fielding BC. Coronavirus envelope protein: current knowledge. Virol J 2019; 16(1): 69. [http://dx.doi.org/10.1186/s12985-019-1182-0] [PMID: 31133031]

[29] Gunathilake KD, Rupasinghe HV. Recent Perspectives on the Medicinal Potential of Chaigne-Delalande B, Li FY, O'Connor GM, Lukacs MJ, Jiang P, Zheng L. Science 2013; 341(6142): 186-91. [PMID: 23846901]

[30] Chattopadhyay D, Ojha D, Mondal S, Goswami D. Validation of antiviral potential of herbal ethnomedicine. 2015. [http://dx.doi.org/10.1016/B978-0-12-800874-4.00008-8]

[31] Chen F, Chan KH, Jiang Y, *et al. In vitro* susceptibility of 10 clinical isolates of SARS coronavirus to selected antiviral compounds. *J. FClin. Virol.*, 2004;31(1)Ginger. Botanics 2015; 5: 55-63.

[32] Chavan R, Shinde P, Girkar K, Madage R, Chowdhary A. Assessment of Anti-Influenza activity and hemagglutination inhibition of *Plumbago indica* and *Allium sativum* extracts. Pharmacognosy Res 2016; 8(2): 105-11. [http://dx.doi.org/10.4103/0974-8490.172562] [PMID: 27034600]

[33] Chen IY, Chang SC, Wu HY, *et al.* Upregulation of the chemokine (C-C motif) ligand 2 *via* a severe acute respiratory syndrome coronavirus spike-ACE2 signaling pathway. J Virol 2010; 84(15): 7703-12.
[http://dx.doi.org/10.1128/JVI.02560-09] [PMID: 20484496]

[34] Cheng L, Zheng W, Li M, *et al.* Citrus fruits are rich in flavonoids for immunoregulation and potential targeting ACE2. Preprints 2020.

[35] Cheng PW, Ng LT, Chiang LC, Lin CC. Antiviral effects of saikosaponins on human coronavirus 229E *in vitro*. Clin Exp Pharmacol Physiol 2006; 33(7): 612-6.
[http://dx.doi.org/10.1111/j.1440-1681.2006.04415.x] [PMID: 16789928]

[36] Chikezie PC, Ibegbulem CO, Mbagwu FN. Bioactive principles from medicinal plants. Res J Phytochem 2015; 9(3): 88-115.
[http://dx.doi.org/10.3923/rjphyto.2015.88.115]

[37] Chiru T, Fursenco C, Ciobanu N, *et al.* Use of medicinal plants in complementary treatment of the common cold and influenza – Perception of pharmacy customers in Moldova and Romania. J Herb Med 2020; 21: 100346.
[http://dx.doi.org/10.1016/j.hermed.2020.100346]

[38] Choi HS, Kim SL, Kim JH, Lee DS. The FDA-approved anti-asthma medicine ciclesonide inhibits lung cancer stem cells through hedgehog signaling-mediated SOX2 regulation. Int J Mol Sci 2020; 21(3): 1014.
[http://dx.doi.org/10.3390/ijms21031014] [PMID: 32033067]

[39] Chowdhury MA, Shahid MA, Kashem MA. Scope of natural plant extract to deactivate COVID-19. Eur PMC 2020; 23: 45-70.

[40] Cinatl J, Morgenstern B, Bauer G, Chandra P, Rabenau H, Doerr HW. Glycyrrhizin, an active component of liquorice roots, and replication of SARS-associated coronavirus. Lancet 2003; 361(9374): 2045-6.
[http://dx.doi.org/10.1016/S0140-6736(03)13615-X] [PMID: 12814717]

[41] Combs Jr, McClung JP. In: Combs, G.F., McClung, J.M (Eds.). Academic press 2016; 1-593.

[42] Coutard B, Valle C, de Lamballerie X, Canard B, Seidah NG, Decroly E. The spike glycoprotein of the new coronavirus 2019-nCoV contains a furin-like cleavage site absent in CoV of the same clade. Antiviral Res 2020; 176(10): 104742.
[http://dx.doi.org/10.1016/j.antiviral.2020.104742] [PMID: 32057769]

[43] Cui J, Li F, Shi ZL. Origin and evolution of pathogenic coronaviruses. Nat Rev Microbiol 2019; 17(3): 181-92.
[http://dx.doi.org/10.1038/s41579-018-0118-9] [PMID: 30531947]

[44] De Clercq E. Selective virus inhibitors. Microbiologica 1990; 13(2): 165-78.
[PMID: 1693749]

[45] De Clercq E. Toward improved anti-HIV chemotherapy: therapeutic strategies for intervention with HIV infections. J Med Chem 1995; 38(14): 2491-517.
[http://dx.doi.org/10.1021/jm00014a001] [PMID: 7543152]

[46] Ding S, Jiang H, Fang J. Regulation of immune function by polyphenols. J Immunol Res 2018; 2018: 1-8.
[http://dx.doi.org/10.1155/2018/1264074] [PMID: 29850614]

[47] Elfiky AA. Natural products may interfere with SARS-CoV-2 attachment to the host cell. J Biomol Struct Dyn 2020; 34: 1-10.
[http://dx.doi.org/10.1080/07391102.2020.1761881] [PMID: 32340551]

[48] Fan Y, Zhao K, Shi ZL, Zhou P. Bat Coronaviruses in China. Viruses 2019; 11(3): 210.
[http://dx.doi.org/10.3390/v11030210] [PMID: 30832341]

[49] Fortunatov MN. EXperimental use of phytoncides for therapeutic and prophylactic purpose. Vopr Pedia Okhrany Materia 1952; 20(2): 55-8.

[50] Gaikwad MS, Meshram BG, Chaugule BB. On occurrence of the genus Porphyridium Nageli: new to *India.* J Algal Biomass Util 2009; 1: 102-6.

[51] Ganjhu RK, Mudgal PP, Maity H, *et al.* Herbal plants and plant preparations as remedial approach for viral diseases. Virusdisease 2015; 26(4): 225-36.
[http://dx.doi.org/10.1007/s13337-015-0276-6] [PMID: 26645032]

[52] Gautret P, Lagier JC, Parola P, *et al.* Hydroxychloroquine and azithromycin as a treatment of COVID-19: results of an open-label non-randomized clinical trial. Int J Antimicrob Agents 2020; 56(1): 105949.
[http://dx.doi.org/10.1016/j.ijantimicag.2020.105949] [PMID: 32205204]

[53] Geresh S, Adin I, Yarmolinsky E, Karpasas M. Characterization of the extracellular polysaccharide of Porphyridium sp.: molecular weight determination and rheological properties. Carbohydr Polym 2002; 50(2): 183-9.
[http://dx.doi.org/10.1016/S0144-8617(02)00019-X]

[54] Ghosh T, Chattopadhyay K, Marschall M, Karmakar P, Mandal P, Ray B. Focus on antivirally active sulfated polysaccharides: From structure–activity analysis to clinical evaluation. Glycobiology 2009; 19(1): 2-15.
[http://dx.doi.org/10.1093/glycob/cwn092] [PMID: 18815291]

[55] Gilani AH, Khan A, Raoof M, *et al.* Gastrointestinal, selective airways and urinary bladder relaxant effects of Hyoscyamus niger are mediated through dual blockade of muscarinic receptors and Ca^{2+} channels. Fundam Clin Pharmacol 2008; 22(1): 87-99.
[http://dx.doi.org/10.1111/j.1472-8206.2007.00561.x] [PMID: 18251725]

[56] Gilca M, Tiplica GS, Salavastru CM. Traditional and ethnobotanical dermatology practices in Romania and other Eastern European countries. Clin Dermatol 2018; 36(3): 338-52.
[http://dx.doi.org/10.1016/j.clindermatol.2018.03.008] [PMID: 29908576]

CHAPTER 7

Herbal Immune-Booster for COVID-19

Raja Chakraborty[1], **Saikat Sen**[2], **Bhargab Jyoti Sahariah**[3], **Chayanika Bordoloi**[4,*] and **Sunil Mistry**[5]

[1] *Institute of Pharmacy, Assam Don Bosco University, Tapesia Gardens, Kamarkuchi, Sonapur, Assam, India*

[2] *Faculty of Pharmaceutical Science, Assam Down Town University, Assam, India*

[3] *NETES Institute of Pharmaceutical Science, Guwahati, Assam, India*

[4] *NEF College of Pharmacy, Guwahati, Assam, India*

[5] *Apex Institute of Pharmacy, Samaspur, Chunar, Mirzapur, UP-231304, India*

Abstract: Medicinal plants always play a vital role by enhancing immunity and protecting us against different infections caused by microorganisms like fungi, bacteria, and viruses. The complex immune protection mechanism produces limitless cells or chemicals to control the spectrum of infectious agents and diseases caused by them. Medicinal plants contain different immunomodulatory constituents that amplify or inhibit the components present in the immune system. In India, people have used numerous medicinal plants and plant products since ancient times to boost the immune system and maintain its normal functioning capacity. Traditional herbaceuticals can boost body defense and improvise our health to survive better. In the last two years, the COVID-19 pandemic became a significant health concern. The healthcare system and scientists are fighting generously to save people. Existing medical facilities are not enough to beat the pandemic condition; therefore, the search for alternative remedies is gaining attention. Indeed, public health measures and the immune-boosting process are considered crucial approaches to dwindle the threat and mortality caused by infection. This chapter highlighted immune boosters from plant sources that can play an essential role as an alternative approaches to managing the current pandemic scenario.

Keywords: Immune System, Medicinal Plant, Herbal Booster, Pandemic, COVID-19.

1. INTRODUCTION

The immune system is an integral part of the body, consisting of complex cellular elements that secrete chemicals to conserve the integrity of the body against

* **Corresponding author Chayanika Bordoloi**: NEF College of Pharmacy, Guwahati, Assam, India; Tel: 9430628231; E-mail: bordoloichayanika15@gmail.com

peripheral infection. The exact function of the immune system is to balance and avoid the incidence of the enormous disorders caused by infectious agents. Immunomodulators can be natural or synthetic substances that can suppress or trigger innate and adaptive immune mechanisms [1].

Infectious diseases are very fast-spreading diseases caused by various microorganisms such as viruses, bacteria, fungi, protists, and other pathogenic agents. Pathogenic agents can cause disease by different disease-spreading conditions like coughing, sneezing, and physical contact. Contaminated water, exchanged body fluids, and droplet contaminations also play important roles in such a process. The innate immune system is the initial or first-line defense of the human body against invading pathogens, nonspecific. The innate immune systems are not activated against any particular pathogen but can provide a total defense. Skin is considered a physical barrier and can exert nonspecific defense against invading pathogens. Enzymes present in saliva, mucus, and tears exert defense by digesting invading microorganisms like bacteria. In response to the pathogen's entry into the body, the innate immune mechanism is activated in the initial stage [2].

Entry and spared of pathogenic microorganisms lead to an inflammatory response as a part of the defense mechanism that causes the flow of white blood cells in infected tissues.White blood cells (phagocytes) include neutrophils and protect us by engulfing and destroying bacteria. The immune system also secretes certain chemicals that maintain the body temperature and induce fever. Fever can slow down orstoppathogen's growth and thus help enhance immune responses in the body. Once pathogens invade our body without responding to innate immune defenses, an adaptive immune response gets activated to defend the same [2].

The primary cells of the immune system are known as lymphocytes and can be divided into two types, *i.e.*, B-lymphocyte cell and T -lymphocyte cell. Bone marrow produces B-lymphocyte cells, and maturation of B-lymphocyte takes place in the bone marrow itself. T-lymphocyte cells are also produced in the bone marrow but mature in the thymus. Humoral immunity is the aspect of immunity that consists of serum antibodies produced by plasma cells and exert their function throughout the body. Humoral immunity begins its action when an antibody of B-lymphocyte cell binds with a pathogen, and B-lymphocyte cell presents the pathogen in front of the helper T cell. Activated B cells also rapidly grow to produce plasma cells, which can release antibodies into the blood. Memory B cells are the specialized cells to store information about the pathogen to have future immunity [3].

2. OUTBREAK OF CORONAVIRUS IN THE 21ST CENTURY

COVID-19 pandemic disease has become a global concern in the 21st century; mortality rises regardless of existing medical facilities [4]. Highly communicable COVID-19 is responsible for a large number of morbidities and mortalities around the globe. Non-availability of vaccines until the early part of 2021 or scarcity of adequate vaccines around the world worsens the situation. In the 21stcentury, viral diseases are becoming more active throughout the world. In the last two decades, the world has witnessed serious infections caused by SARS-CoV, MERS-CoV, and different influenza viruses [5]. In the present scenario, COVID-19 can be considered the world's 3rd most dangerous disease for humans, spreading very fast to all parts of the world. Reports showed that approximately 213 countries are infected with coronavirus [6]. Experts confirmed its clinical characteristics, and it is pretty similar to a pneumonia condition. In March 2020, the World Health Organisation (WHO) announced COVID-19 as a pandemic [7]. COVID-19 disease is caused by the virus named SARS-CoV-2, coined by the International Committee on Taxonomy of Viruses [7]. SARS-CoV has sequence homology with the bat coronavirus and spike glycoproteins present in the virus of SARS play an important role in invading and transmitting the infection from human to human [8]. The spreading capacity of the novel coronavirus and its diagnosis are relatively different from the SARS-CoV virus. The nucleotide patterns of the SARS-CoV virus and their receptor binding sites are unique [9].

The government, WHO, and other healthcare organizations are working together to stop the spread of viral infection. Minimizing the physical contact, isolation, and screening of infected people during the initial stages of infection and sanitization are vital approaches to control the spread of COVID-19. The viral infection can transmit from person to person through the saliva or nose discharge of an infected patient. Manufacturing industries are producing tonnes of masks, and sanitizers to prevent or control the situation [10]. Drugs are in the clinical trial stage, and no specific medicines are available to treat the disease condition yet. Some existing drugs available in the market, like Lopinavir, Chloroquine, Nitazoxanide, Ritonavir, *etc.*, are used to reduce disease progression and balance the virusload [7].

It was observed that COVID-19 virus infection develops in people with weak immune systems, such as older people or people with comorbidities. Certain beneficial bacteria that live in our gut protect us against a spectrum of diseases. The growth of beneficial intestinal bacteria can be increased through the intake of healthy plant-based foods. According to WHO, the COVID-19 virus is similar to different coronavirus types in morphological and chemical compositions [11]. New strains of COVID-19 became a challenge for the healthcare system. It was also reported that COVID-19 could be spared as a droplet transmission from person to person. Infection of COVID-19 can also spread when a person touches the contaminated surface and then touches the eyes, nose, or mouth [12, 13]. SARS-CoV-2 infection can be classified into three phases: the first phase is known as the asymptomatic phase, the second phase is known as the non-severe symptomatic phase, and the third phase is known as the severe symptomatic phase [14]. A few patients are progressing to a severe stage of infection, *i.e.*, the third phase, and they use to suffer from multiorgan failure in the end stage [15]. The SARS-CoV-2 virus enters the host's body and binds to ACE2 receptors, which results in the initiation of immune responses. In SARS-CoV-2 infection, both innate and adaptive immune responses are activated to protect our bodies [5]. In comparison to non-severe patients, critically severe patients' blood serum contains elevated biomarkers such as TNF-α, IL-2, IL-6, IL-7, IL-8, IL- 10, GCSF, MCP1, and MIP1-alpha, which result in cytokinin strom [16 - 18].

3. TRADITIONAL MEDICINE IN CORONA PANDEMIC

Chinese medicines and Ayurvedic medicines are choices of remedies throughout the globe with a vast capacity to reduce the severity of diseases caused by viruses since ancient times (1500-500 BCE) [19, 20]. The Ayurvedic medicine system is considered one of the oldest systems of medicine globally, and it can manage a wide range of ailments with no or little side effects. This system of medicine is well known for different treatment procedures to cure multiple disorders [21]. Ayurvedic science is well equipped with the knowledge of various microorganisms and their infective capacity to create any disease condition [22]. Both the Ayurvedic and Siddha systems originate from different parts of India and are very extensively used by other people of India to cure significant ailments, including diseases caused by microorganisms [23]. Plants play a central role in Ayurvedic and Sidha medicine. Identification and isolation of bioactive constituents present in the plants and screening of effectiveness might help manage deadly infections in a better way. We can rely on ancient medicinal plants that are the source of key phytomolecules to boost our immunity or with antiviral activity [24]. Traditional Chinese medicine (TCM) also includes different herbs for curing various ailments. Over 10,000 herbal plants or plant products are included in TCM, and such medicines are prevalent in China and contain a large pool of plants with immunomodulatory activity [25]. TCM system has been used widely in China to manage the SARS epidemic since 2003. This system plays an essential role in treating and preventing many outbreak diseases in China since ancient times. Many plant-based immunity-boosting herbs are available around us, such as garlic, black cumin, licorice, cinnamon, *etc.*, that are well reported in various traditional medicines. The inclusion of those herbs in our diet as tea or as food will boost immunity.

In India, to control the COVID-19 pandemic, the Ministry of AYUSH includes different traditional medicines available under ayurvedic, Yoga and Naturopathy, Unani, Siddha, and Homeopathy. They suggested drinking Kadha as an immune booster to reduce tenderness during COVID-19 infection [26]. Kadha is an extract prepared from many spices and herbs available commonly in India. Traditional healthcare professionals of India generally recommend classical Ayurvedic medicines to manage infectious diseases. AYUSH-64 is one of the Ayurvedic medicines that can cure malaria and other fevers. An Ayurvedic formulation prepared of sushi (*Zingiber officinale* Roscoe.), Lavagna (*Syzygium aromaticum*), and maricha (*Piper nigrum*) have been prescribed to healthy people as well as COVID-19 infected persons. This formulation is used as an immune booster to support humoral and cell-mediated immune responses against viral infections and reduce hyper-responsiveness of the airway and nasal blockage [27 - 29]. In Ayurveda formulations, ghee is the main fatty acid component for upregulating the resistance [30].

AYUSH has recommended some medicinal plants for prophylactic action against COVID-19. *Tinospora cordifolia*, *Andrographi spaniculata*, *Cydonia oblonga Zizyphus jujube* and *Cordiamyxa, Arsenicum album* are found effective against SARS-CoV-2 as immune-modulators. The symptomatic phase of COVID-19 infection can be treated with Agastya Haritaki and prevent upper respiratory tract infections. Anuthaila is a sesame oil drop that can cure respiratory infections during COVID-19 infection [23].

Adhatoda vasica extract was found to reduce enhanced inflammation of the airway. *Adhatoda vasica* extract reduces TGF-β1, IL-6, HIF-1α levels and recovers the mice's overall survival rates, and rescues the siRNA-induced inflammation and associated blood coagulation. *Adhatoda vasica* causes the downregulation of hypoxia, inflammatory condition, TGF-β1, angiogenesis genes, and upregulation of the genes related to adaptive immunity [31]. Spices rich in antioxidant and immunomodulatory phytochemicals can be a potential source of natural substances against COVID-19. Several clinical trials of Ayurvedic formulation against COVID-19 are in process, and different spices like *Curcuma longa*, *Cinnamomum zeylanicum*, *Ocimum sanctum*, *Elettaria cardamomum, Cinnamomum tamala*, *Piper longum*, *Tinospora cordifolia*, and *Zingiber officinale* are the key components of those formulations [32]. The therapeutic potential of extracts of Tea (*C. Sinensis*) and Haritaki (*T. chebula)* against SARS-CoV-2 based on $3CL^{pro}$ protease activity inhibition was reported.

4. PLANT BASED-IMMUNITY BOOSTER FOR COVID-19

Naturally occurring products and phytomedicines are becoming an essential source of medicine and increasing their demand worldwide. These naturally occurring products are getting more important in society globally. People have started believing in different ways of drug formulations because they face chronic and lifestyle-related disorders nowadays. They are serious about improving lifestyles and minimizing disorders [33]. In ancient times, herbal medicines were the only choice for healing any disease condition. Evidence showed that different herbal formulations are in use for decades as antiviral products. However, in such a process, it is essential to understand the infective capacity of the virus and how herbs can prevent infection, stop virus life-cycle and replication, retard viral assembly and release conditions. Traditional medicines have a high safety profile and clinical characteristics, so there is a gradual increase in the acceptance of herbal medicine [34]. Chemical drugs have a high level of side effects on the human body, but herbal therapy has high effectiveness with minimal side effects. The World Health Organization has also acknowledged that herbal therapies are effective, and approximately 80% of the world's population has trust in such medicines [26].

Research works are trying to find the treatment of coronavirus infection using medicinal plants. Preclinical studies on experimental animals indicated that different plant species such as *Indigo feratinctoria*, *Gymnema sylvestre*, *Evolvulus alsinoides*, *Vitextrifolia*, *Allium sativum*, *Pergularia demi*, *Clerodendrum ineme*, *Leucas aspera, Abutilon indicum*, *Clitoria tematea*, *Sphaeranthus indicus*, and *Cassia alata* could be effective against SARS-CoV [35]. In Asia, mountains are flooded with varieties of plants with a high degree of medicinal value to treat a range of respiratory infections [36]. *Hyoscyamus niger*, *Cynara scolymus*, *Verbascum thapsus*, *Justicia adhatoda, and Cynara scolymus* are the medicinal plants that are effective on the SARS-CoV-2 virus. These plants also showed activity against the influenza virus which act by inhibiting Ca^{2+} channels [37]. Different plants such as *Coriandrum sativum*, *Boerhaavia diffusa, Punica granatum*, *Cassia occidentalis*, *Embeliaribes, and Coscinium fenestratum* have shown their effectivity on ACE receptors [38, 39]. *Salacia oblonga* is an important plant that inhibits angiotensin II which is related to bronchitis conditions and lung disorders. Herbal plants used previously to treat HIV can also be considered suitable agents to treat COVID-19 infection. Some medicinal plants such as *Acacia nilotica*, *Eugenia jambolana*, *Ocimum sanctum*, *Euphorbia granulate*, *Vitex negundo*, *Ocimum kikim*, *Solanum nigrum*, *Ocimum scharicum*, *etc.* have effectivity on HIV treatment and can also be considered a potent agent for SARS-CoV-2 treatment [40 - 43]. The plant *Sambucus ebulus* also inhibits the growth of the enveloped virus, and it will be studied further as a target against this virus [44].

Constituents isolated from medicinal plants can be used to activate the immune system. Herbal formulations using such medicinal plants can be designed against COVID-19 infection. Some important phytoconstituents like cannabinoid, glycyrrhizic acid, hesperidin, carrageenan, lepidine E, curcumin, nigelledine, sanguiin, protocatechuic acid, 6-gingerol, naringin, fraxetin, capsaicin, limonene, oleanolic acid, eugenol, piperine, quercetin, withaferin, flavanones, baicalein, ginkgolic acid, allyl disulfide, galangin, myricitrin, nictoflorin, aloesin, apigenin, epicatechingallate, ginkgolide A, silybin, rutin, apiin, jensenone, herbaceous, sitosterol, betulinic acid, carvacrol, chlorogenic acid, gallic acid, thymol, santalic acid, *etc.* are the prime target of research against the viral infection [45]. Secondary metabolites are very useful constituents of plants, and they have an active role in preventing diseases. Many important secondary metabolites such as terpenoids, polyphenols, flavonoids, dipeptides, and polysaccharides can play a potent role against viral and other microbial infections.

4.1. Terpenoids

Triterpenes are the chemical components present in plant species, composed of 6 isoprene units in their chemical structure [46]. Terpenoids play a vital role in cell metabolism, sterol biosynthesis, and biological activity against viruses. The primary therapeutic strategy to cure viral infection is to identify the plant products having specific enzyme inhibitory effects. Terpenoids are a very common and important secondary metabolite found in more than 36,000 plant species [47].

Recently, it has been reported that the structure of terpenoid constituents resembles the protease of COVID-19 virus, which was found from different types of databases available such as PubChem, Protein Data Bank (PDB), *etc.* Some sophisticated molecular docking techniques are used to find out the protein structure using MVD (molegro virtual dockers) software. Terpenoids were isolated from different plants *e.g.* Salvinorin A derived from *Salvia divinorum*, citral derived from *Backhousia citriodora*, Bilobalide and Ginkgolide A derived from *Gingko biloba*, Noscapine derived from the plants of Papaveraceae family, menthol derived from Mentha, Beta Selinene derived from *Apium graveolens* plants and Forskolin derived from *Plectranthus barbatus* [46, 47].

4.2. Polyphenols and Flavonoids

Polyphenols are commonly present in plants with a range of therapeutic activities. Polyphenols can increase immunity and involve the destruction of foreign substances. Generally, polyphenols accumulate in the cell through different receptors, resulting in the activation of the signaling pathways and immunity [48]. Some scientists in 2020 conducted an *in-silico* study on natural polyphenols and identified that some polyphenols could inhibit COVID-19 protease (Mpro) capable of controlling the disease. A docking study with 80 different types of flavonoids indicated that compounds like rutin, apiin, diosmin, hesperidin, diacetyl curcumin, *etc.* have an inhibitory effect against COVID-19 infection [48, 49].

Flavonoids are important secondary metabolites found in different plant species, and are active against the viral infection [49]. Flavonoids are the secondary metabolites and are the important constituents of plants. They are one of the most important polyphenols present in the human diet. Different naturally occurring flavonoids such as naringin, quercetin, catechin, and hesperetin have their activity against respiratory syncytial virus, HSV-1, poliovirus type-1, and parainfluenza virus type 3. It was observed that glycyrrhizin reduces SARS-Cov infection. *In-silico* study showed that glycyrrhizin is a potential inhibitor of COVID-19 [34].

4.3. Dipeptides for COVID-19

Chymotrypsin is a biologically active compound with similar activity to protease enzyme, and it is already proved that it has an inhibitory effect on coronavirus. Recently, a total of 31 molecules in India have been identified, which can be utilized as protease inhibitors against the COVID-19 virus. Aurantiamide is a dipeptide, a plant-derived biologically active compound extracted from the plant *Piper aurantiacum*. Aurantiamide acetate has diverse therapeutic potentials against many ailments, such as anti-cancer and anti-inflammatory activity along with its antiviral activity [50]. Except for aurantiamide, many other potentially active plant peptides have an important role in recovering from COVID-19 infection [51].

4.4. Polysaccharides for Immunity

Polysaccharides found in plants are structurally diverse biomolecules than the other phytochemicals and have many applications in medicine and pharmaceutical sciences [52]. Polysaccharides can be isolated from different plant parts such as cell walls, tree exudates, seeds, roots, and animal sources such as chondroitin sulfate, chitin, and hyaluronan. Several bacteria and fungi have hydrocolloids in their structures like well, xanthan and gellan. They are an important source of naturally occurring polysaccharides [53]. Another important polysaccharide resource is algae *i.e.* mucopolysac charides. The storage polysaccharides are largely extracted from the algae [53]. Polysaccharides are found naturally in plants and are the richest source of structural and functional biopolymers. Polysaccharides present in plants have been reported for different bioactivities like anti-tumor, anti-coagulant, antiviral, and immunomodulatory activity. A polysaccharide has specific inhibitory activity against different viruses. Giloya herb contains diterpene compounds and polysaccharides with immunomodulatory and adaptogenic activity. Giloya herbal extract was studied and revealed that it can enhance IgG antibodies in the serum and activate macrophages and B cell-mediated immunity [54].

4.5. Vitamin D Rich Foods

Vitamin D is helpful for the immune system and indirectly inhibits the risk of infection [55]. Vitamin D3 is formed within the skin by interacting with UV radiation and forming 7-dehydrocholesterol in a heat-generating reaction. The importance of vitamin D comes from the compound calcitriol, which can pass through receptors to enter the nucleus. Vitamin D can be utilized in several ways to prevent the risk of viral infection and mortality rate. Vitamin D is important for joints and junctions which can help to promote junctions of tight, gap junctions and adherent junctions. Studies revealed that viruses can able to damage the integrity of junctions. Vitamin D also helps to improve the innate immunity of our body. Vitamin D is useful for cellular defense in a normal individual by modulating the level of cytokine biomarkers. Generally, in COVID-19 patients, secretion of inflammatory and pro-inflammatory cytokines increases in the response of viral infections [55].

4.6. Vitamin C and E Rich Foods to Induce Immunity

Vitamin C is a necessary component for kids, adults, and elderly people to improve their systems system. Fruits are a rich source of vitamin C such as orange, kiwi, papaya, and guava should be included in the daily diet to improve immunity. Many green vegetables like bell peppers, eggplant, spinach, beetroots, and cauliflower are considered rich sources of vitamin C. Other vegetables such as mushrooms and broccoli have a few immune-boosting activities and could be included in the diet. Elderly people can also take Spirulina and Curcumin in their diet as they are rich in vitamin C and minerals. Vitamin C is a water-soluble vitamin and very useful for the treatment of sepsis and septic shock. These conditions can be life-threatening and result from inflammation produced by any pathogenic microorganisms [56].

Vitamin E has a vital role in maintaining the overall health and immunity of older adults. It is a powerful antioxidant and can protect the body from various infections by bacteria, and viruses. Soaked almonds, peanut butter, sunflower seeds, and even hazelnuts are rich sources of vitamin E. Vitamin E works physiologically in unspecific ways and inhibits lipid peroxidation. Vitamin E is usually helpful as a radical peroxyl scavenger and it can protect the polyunsaturated fats of plasma membranes. Vitamin E has a prominent activity for preserving immune responses and activating humoral and cell-mediated immunity [57, 58].

4.6.1. Vitamin A

Vitamin A is an essential constituent of food and fat-soluble vitamin. It has an important role in regulating vision, growth of body and maturity, and protecting the mucosal layer and epithelium layer of the human body [59]. Vitamin A has potent immunomodulatory activity in the functioning of humoral and cellular immune responses. Various plant-based sources of vitamin A are broccoli, mushroom, amla, carrot, avocado, almond, citrus, guava, *etc.*, and play an important role in preventing COVID-19 infection by modelinghumoral and cellular immune response. A wide range of minerals, probiotics, and nutraceuticals are also observed to be effective for viral infections and can stimulate immune activity [60, 61].

4.6.2. Minerals

Zinc and magnesium are essential micronutrients useful in DNA synthesis and cell proliferation [62]. They are also involved in regulating innate and adaptive immune responses, cell signaling, and the production of immune cells. Zinc-containing foods can include red meat and shellfish . Magnesium is also an important mineral to improve the immune response, the electrolyte can help the body by strengthening the immune cells such as NK cells, lymphocyte cells, *etc.* Minerals are also involved in the production of energy for cells known as adenosine triphosphate (ATP). Magnesium is the vital element of hemoglobin present in blood cells. They have a responsibility to deliver oxygen throughout the body. Magnesium is a crucial element for COVID-19 infection because the virus especially affects the body's respiratory system and alters the oxygen supply through blood. Magnesium mineral-rich foods are black beans, dark chocolates, avocados, whole grains, *etc* [63].

Trace elements like copper have a vital role in the growth, development, and division of immune cells. Selenium is another important trace element with a broad range of anti-inflammatory activities, antioxidant activity, *etc.*, and is also used as a supplement [64, 65]. Plant-based foods like beans, grains, nuts, mushrooms, peanuts, cereals, garlic, lentils, *etc.* have a spectrum of minerals in them, and these foods are required to be included in the diet during the COVID-19 protocol.

4.7. Nutraceuticals Supplements and Probiotics for Immunity

Nutraceuticals are considered food for physiological assistance and they are sometimes important to protect against different spectrums of diseases. We can consider a wide range of products under nutraceuticals such as genetically engineered foods, dietary supplements, processed cereals, isolated nutrients, beverages, soups, *etc* [66]. From previous studies, it was found that some nutraceuticals can enhance immune functions. In their studies, McCarty and Di Nicolantonio concluded that nutraceuticals can reduce the symptoms of diseases and provide protection against coronavirus and influenza infection. Another important product is probiotics, which are live microorganisms, present in different parts of our body, especially the intestine, to produce beneficial health effects. They are also involved in the activation of specific immunity by the synthesis of antibodies. Akatsu and his group have conducted a study in 2013 and reported that *Bifidobacterium longum* microbe has an immunomodulatory effect as a supplement of the immune responses in an older person. It was observed that lactobacilli probiotics can reduce cold and pharyngeal symptoms [67].

5. INDIAN SPICES APPLICABLE AS AN IMMUNE BOOSTER

In India, people consume a significant amount of spices every day as part of their diet. Normally, people consume spices mixed with hot water, milk, ghee, and cooked food. Daily intake of some important spices as a part of a regular diet can help to develop and strengthen the immune system. Researchers proved that spices are helpful in inducing both innate and adaptive immunity of the human body. It was observed that spices were used to treat cancer, brain disorders, antiviral, immunity disorders, *etc.* One of the essential spices generally used by Indians is turmeric, and a recent study showed that turmeric can control the COVID-19 infection [68]. In the time of pandemic situation, Govt. of India also promoted herbal spices and their use in diet to boost the immune system that can help the body fight against COVID-19 infection. Spices can regulate the inflammation process and also inhibit the release of excess cytokines. They have also exerted antioxidant activity which is essential for normal health. Therefore, the infection prevention nature of spices is well established, and these can play an important role in averting COVID-19 infection by activating innate and adaptive immunity. Some important Indian spices are Asafoetida, Cardamom, Coriander,

Cinnamon, Capsicum, Ginger, Garlic, Turmeric, Fenugreek, Mustard, Fennel, Ajwain, Black pepper, Clove, Cuminum, *etc* (Table **1**) [69].

Table 1. Potential spice with immunomodulatory, antiviral, or anti-inflammatory activity [32, 70, 71].

Sl No	Scientific Name and Family	Common Name	Description
1	*Trachyspermum ammi*	Ajwain, Caraway, Carom	Ajwain is used for cold and cough as an expectorant, decongestion, and removal of mucous. Medicinally it is used as antifungal, antinociceptive, antioxidant, antimicrobial, hypolipidemic, cytotoxic, antihypertensive, antispasmodic, nematicidal, antilithiasis, diuretic, antifilarial, anthelmintic, abortifacient, and antitussive agents. The seed contains 2-4.4% oil, which contains thymol used in gastrointestinal bronchial problems and exhibits fungicidal, antimicrobial activity.
2	*Ferula asafoetida*	Asafoetida, Heeng,	It shows carminative, expectorant, antispasmodic, anthelmintic, and aphrodisiac properties. Phytoconstituent exhibited activity against influenza A virus (H1N1) in an *in-vitro* study
3	*Ocimum sanctum*	Tulsi, Basil	One important medicinal herb exhibited antibacterial, antiviral, antifungal, antimalarial, antiprotozoal, anthelmintic, anti-inflammatory, antioxidant, analgesic, antiallergic, immunomodulatory, antistress, and much other pharmacological activities. Basil was found to enhance T cell and NK cell levels which fight against the viral infection.
4	*Allium sativum*	Lasan, Garlic	Garlic boosts the immune system by enhancing and protecting the immune cell against the virus. Allicin and enzyme alliinase were found to possess antiviral activity that causes the common cold and viral pneumonia such as influenza B virus, *Cytomegalovirus*, herpes simplex virus, and human rhinovirus type 2, parainfluenza virus Type 3. Raw garlic is used as cardioprotective, lowering blood pressure and blood cholesterol levels.
6	*Mentha Piperita*	Peppermint, pudina	Peppermint exhibits cytotoxic, antiviral, antibacterial, antioxidant, and antiallergenic activity. It possibly enhances innate immunity that is helpful against respiratory virus infection. Essential oil of peppermint reduced nitric oxide, IL-6, and PGE2 generation in macrophages. It also decreases cellular infection and inflammation.
7	*Zingiber officinale*	Ginger, Adrak	It shows antiviral activity against the human respiratory syncytial virus (HRSV). Fresh ginger inhibits HRSV-induced plaque formation by blocking viral attachment and internalization in both HEp-2 and A549 cell lines. Gingerols and zingerone are the two main phytoconstituents found to inhibit virus replication and stop entering the virus in host cells.

(Table 1) cont.....

Sl No	Scientific name and Family	Common Name	Description
8	*Cinnamomum verum, Cinnamomum zeylanicum*	Cinnamon, Dalchini	Cinnamon prevents throat infections for regular use. It possesses antimicrobial, antifungal, antiviral, antioxidant, antihypertensive, antitumor, antidiabetic, antilipemic, immunomodulatory, and gastroprotective effects. Cinnamon showed an immunomodulatory, antioxidant, and anti-inflammatory effect. It suppresses the expression of cyclooxygenase-2 and MHC I and induces dendritic cells that generate proinflammatory cytokines in low quantity.
9	*Piper longum* Linn.	Black pepper, Kali mirch	Traditionally used as an immune enhancer for treating cold and cough and it gives a relief from sinusitis and nasal congestion. Quercetin is found in black pepper that possesses antiviral and antibacterial properties. Piperine showed the antioxidative, chemoprotective, and anti-apoptotic effect.
10	*Curcuma longa*	Turmeric, haldi	Curcumin was found to possess reno-protective, cardioprotective, anti-inflammatory, antioxidant, antiviral, antibacterial, antifungal, immunomodulatory activity. Curcumin was found to increase mucosal CD4(+) T-cells and B-cells in animals. It also inhibits different pro-inflammatory cytokinin.
11	*Capsicum annuum*	Capsicum	Capsicum extract and capsaicin-producing immunomodulatory activity were also found to reduce the production of IL-2, interferon-γ, IL-4, and IL-5, and reduction in CD3 cells and enhancement of CD-19 cells. Capsicum modulates the T-cell immune response. Capsaicin promoted the activation of dendritic cells that are related to immunomodulatory activity, it suppressed both T-cell receptor-dependent and production of IL-2. Capsicum exhibited anti-inflammatory activity.
12	*Elettaria cardamomum*	Cardamom, elaichi	Cardamom showed antioxidant, immunomodulatory, and anti-inflammatory activity. An experimental study showed that cardamom enhances lymphocyte, white blood, CD4+, and CD8+ cells and can be developed as immunostimulating agents.
13	*Coriandrum sativum*	Coriander, dhaniya	Coriander exhibited antioxidant, anti-tumor, antifungal, and antimicrobial activity. Coriander also exhibited anti-inflammatory and analgesic activity.
14	*Trigonella foenum-graecum*	Fenugreek	It showed antioxidant, antidiabetic, hepatoprotective, immunomodulatory, and anti-inflammatory activity. In experimental animals, the extract of fenugreek reduced the levels of IL-1a, IL-1b, IL-2, IL-6, and TNF-α.
15	*Syzygium aromaticum*	Clove, long	Clove exhibited antioxidant, anti-inflammatory, analgesic, and antidiabetic activity. It also inhibits bacterial infection and exhibits an antimicrobial effect.

5.1. Herbal Formulations for COVID-19

Traditional medicine professionals recommend many herbal formulations according to the situation or condition of the patient. The therapeutic regimen consists of two different phases, one is medicine, and the second is diet. Different herbal medicinal formulations used to treat the symptoms of COVID-19 infection are Sudarsana Churna, Talisadi Churna, Dhanwantara Gutika, Vidaryadi Ghritam, *etc.* and with these, the patient should maintain a healthy diet [72]. Some other Ayurvedic formulations are used to treat symptoms of COVID-19 infection which are Pathyadikwatha, Lakshmi vilasa rasa, Shadangathoya, Panavyoshadivati, Nishamalakikwatha, Nagaradikwatha, Sudarshana Ghana vati, Vasa swarasa, Guduchiswarasa, Kantakarichurna, Saindhava, Gojihvadikwatha, Dashamularishta, Agastya rasayana, Haridrakhanda, Kumaryasava, Talisadichurna, *etc* [73].

In China, many herbal formulations are used in the symptomatic treatment of COVID-19 infection, such as Sang BeiZhisou San, Jia Jian Zhengqi San, Da Yuan Yin, Shen Shu San, Huo Po Xia Ling Tang, Qingwen Baidu Yin, Sheng Jiang San, Jing Fang Baidu San, JiuweiQianghuo pill, Yin Qiao Sam, Sang Ju Yin, *etc.* Korean traditional medicine system has also published two guidelines for the treatment regimen of COVID-19 infection. In these guidelines, they have segregated the herbal treatment according to the symptoms *i.e.*, severe or mild condition [74].

Researchers and traditional healthcare professionals have already found some important herbs that can be used as preventive and symptomatic treatment of COVID-19. However, further search is going on to find new molecules from herbal sources that can effectively manage the viral infection. Research to find the effectiveness of the traditional formulations used from ancient times to treat viral infection is going on against COVID-19 infection.

6. CHALLENGES, POTENTIAL SOLUTIONS, AND FUTURE PROSPECTS

In the COVID-19 pandemic, all the developed countries are also suffering equally with the developing countries. Even the most developed country like the USA, is also suffering seriously. The advanced developed technologies are being used to manage the situation effectively. Health professionals are working hard to save patients' lives. The situation is sudden and very much challenging to the globe and global communities. Even though different pharmaceutical companies are manufacturing different vaccines, it is also not possible to prevent the disease completely in the current situation. Different antiviral and other supplements are in use to treat the symptoms of the disease. Tocilizumab is a monoclonal antibody and other such drugs found beneficial to suppress the cytokinin strom in severe patients. Nevertheless, boosting immunity and preventing infection are essential to avert further complications caused by COVID-19.

Most developing countries use herbal medicines as a primary health care treatment because of their easy availability and negligible side effects. There are several herbal formulations available to treat the symptoms of viral infections and enhance the immune system. There is no specific drug to treat COVID-19; therefore, relying on traditional systems, mainly herbal medicine, to enhance immunity is important. Researchers are working vigorously to find effective medicines from herbs to completely cure COVID-19 because there are infinite important herbs available to treat viral infections and induce the immunity system. Traditional medicine systems such as the Ayurvedic system, Unani system, and Siddha system have suggested symptomatic remedies against COVID-19 infection. Different herbal formulations, plant-based medicines, extracts/decoction, and crude drugs are the choice of medicine to boost immunity and create a difference in our fight against COVID-19. Many plant sources are available in India, showing antiviral activity that can be screened for their effectiveness against COVID-19. Effective medicinal formulations from the herbal source could be helpful to avert the COVID-19 pandemic through their immune-boosting, antioxidant and antiviral properties.

CONCLUSION

The utilization of herbal medicine in the modern era is increasing day by day because of its efficacy and good safety profile. Foods rich in vitamins, minerals, antioxidants, and nutritional properties can boost immunity to fight against infectious diseases. Natural products and phytochemicals have an extensive track record of treating respiratory infections and as immune-boosting agents, and many of them have been approved as a drug. Extensive research and clinical trials aim to target herbal products' capacity to manage COVID-19 infections and post-infectious complications. Progression of COVID-19 results in a cytokine storm, and anti-inflammatory herbs and phytochemicals may be helpful to minimize such life-threatening conditions. It is observed that people's dependency on herbal medicines has increased, and the use of herbal supplements as immune boosters and antioxidants is rising. In this COVID-19 era, practitioners and researchers are looking towards herbal medicines as an alternative to allopathic medicine or as an adjuvant to antiviral drugs and monoclonal antibodies. Research on herbal immune-booster is challenging but has a wide scope to address the COVID-19 pandemic in a better way. Keeping in view the immune-boosting potential of traditional medicines and medicinal plants, appropriate strategies with advanced research targeting promising therapeutic leads to find their mechanism and clinical outcomes are important to uphold the general utility of such medicine.

CONSENT FOR PUBLICATION

Not Applicable.

CONFLICT OF INTEREST

The author declares no conflict of interest, financial or otherwise.

ACKNOWLEDGEMENTS

Declared none.

REFERENCES

[1] McClave SA, Lowen CC, Snider HL. Immunonutrition and enteral hyperalimentation of critically ill patients. Dig Dis Sci 1992; 37(8): 1153-61. [http://dx.doi.org/10.1007/BF01296554] [PMID: 1499437]

[2] Watson RR. Nutrition, immunomodulation, and AIDS: an overview. J Nutr 1992; 122 (Suppl. 3): 715. [http://dx.doi.org/10.1093/jn/122.suppl_3.715]

[3] McMurray DN, Bartow RA. Immunosuppression and alteration of resistance to pulmonary tuberculosis in guinea pigs by protein undernutrition. J Nutr 1992; 122(3) (Suppl. 3): 738-43. [http://dx.doi.org/10.1093/jn/122.suppl_3.738] [PMID: 1347317]

[4] Ahmad A, Rehman MU, Alkharfy KM. An alternative approach to minimize the risk of coronavirus (Covid-19) and similar infections. Eur Rev Med Pharmacol Sci 2020; 24(7): 4030-4. [PMID: 32329879]

[5] Čivljak R, Markotić A, Kuzman I. The third coronavirus epidemic in the third millennium: what's next? Croat Med J 2020; 61(1): 1-4. [http://dx.doi.org/10.3325/cmj.2020.61.1] [PMID: 32118371]

[6] Acharya KP. Resource poor countries ought to focus on early detection and containment of novel corona virus at the point of entry. Clin Epidemiol Glob Health 2020; 1: 1-2. [http://dx.doi.org/10.1016/j.cegh.2020.03.001] [PMID: 32292836]

[7] Gautret P, Lagier JC, Parola P, *et al.* Hydroxychloroquine and azithromycin as a treatment of COVID-19: results of an open-label non-randomized clinical trial. Int J Antimicrob Agents 2020; 56(1): 105949. [http://dx.doi.org/10.1016/j.ijantimicag.2020.105949] [PMID: 32205204]

[8] Guo YR, Cao QD, Hong ZS, *et al.* The origin, transmission and clinical therapies on coronavirus disease 2019 (COVID-19) outbreak – an update on the status. Mil Med Res 2020; 7(1): 11. [http://dx.doi.org/10.1186/s40779-020-00240-0] [PMID: 32169119]

[9] Wan Y, Shang J, Graham R, Baric RS, Li F. Receptor recognition by the novel coronavirus from Wuhan: an analysis based on decade-long structural studies of SARS coronavirus. J Virol 2020; 94(7): e00127-20. [http://dx.doi.org/10.1128/JVI.00127-20] [PMID: 31996437]

[10] Balachandar V, Mahalaxmi I, Kaavya J, *et al.* COVID-19: emerging protective measures. Eur Rev Med Pharmacol Sci 2020; 24(6): 3422-5. [PMID: 32271461]

[11] World Health Organization (WHO). Coronavirus disease 2019.https://www.who.int/docs/default-source/coronaviruse/situation-reports/20200417-sitrep-88-covid

[12] Peng X, Xu X, Li Y, Cheng L, Zhou X, Ren B. Transmission routes of 2019-nCoV and controls in dental practice. Int J Oral Sci 2020; 12(1): 9. [http://dx.doi.org/10.1038/s41368-020-0075-9] [PMID: 32127517]

[13] Morawska L, Cao J. Airborne transmission of SARS-CoV-2: The world should face the reality. Environ Int 2020; 139: 105730. [http://dx.doi.org/10.1016/j.envint.2020.105730] [PMID: 32294574]

[14] Shi Y, Wang Y, Shao C, *et al.* COVID-19 infection: the perspectives on immune responses. Cell Death Differ 2020; 27(5): 1451-4. [http://dx.doi.org/10.1038/s41418-020-0530-3] [PMID: 32205856]

[15] Cao X. COVID-19: immunopathology and its implications for therapy. Nat Rev Immunol 2020; 20(5): 269-70. [http://dx.doi.org/10.1038/s41577-020-0308-3] [PMID: 32273594]

[16] Huang C, Wang Y, Li X, *et al.* Clinical features of patients infected with 2019 novel coronavirus in Wuhan, China. Lancet 2020; 395(10223): 497-506. [http://dx.doi.org/10.1016/S0140-6736(20)30183-5] [PMID: 31986264]

[17] Qin C, Zhou L, Hu Z, *et al.* Dysregulation of immune response in patients with COVID- 19 in Wuhan, China. Clin Infect Dis 2020; 71(15): 762-8. [http://dx.doi.org/10.1093/cid/ciaa248] [PMID: 32161940]

[18] Wang F, Hou H, Luo Y, *et al.* The laboratory tests and host immunity of COVID-19 patients with different severity of illness. JCI Insight 2020; 5(10): e137799. [http://dx.doi.org/10.1172/jci.insight.137799] [PMID: 32324595]

[19] Chattopadhyay D, Ojha D, Mondal S, Goswami D. Validation of the antiviral potential of herbal ethnomedicine. Evidence-based validation of herbal medicine. Elsevier Public Health Care Collection 2015; 1: 175-200.

[20] Jadhav P, Kapoor N, Thomas B, Lal H, Kshirsagar N. Antiviral potential of selected Indian medicinal (ayurvedic) plants against Herpes Simplex Virus 1 and 2. N Am J Med Sci 2012; 4(12): 641-7. [http://dx.doi.org/10.4103/1947-2714.104316] [PMID: 23272307]

[21] Goothy SSK, Goothy S, Choudhary A, *et al.* Ayurveda's holistic lifestyle approach for the management of coronavirus disease (COVID-19): possible role of Tulsi. Int. J. Res. Pharm. Sci. 2020; (SPL1): 16-8.

[22] Panda AK. Current status of infectious diseases in Ayurveda. Ayursurabhi 2005; 2005: 66-7.

[23] Vellingiri B, Jayaramayya K, Iyer M, *et al.* COVID-19: A promising cure for the global panic. Sci Total Environ 2020; 725: 138277. [http://dx.doi.org/10.1016/j.scitotenv.2020.138277] [PMID: 32278175]

[24] Luo H, Tang QL, Shang YX, *et al.* Can Chinese medicine be used for prevention of coronavirus disease 2019 (COVID-19)? A review of historical classics, research evidence, and current prevention programs. Chin J Integr Med 2020; 1: 1-8.

[25] Lin LL, Shan JJ, Xie T, *et al.* Application of traditional Chinese medical herbs in prevention and treatment of the respiratory syncytial virus. Evidence.-. Based Complementary Altern Med 2016; 2016: 1-14.

[26] 2020.pib.gov.in/PressReleasePage.aspx?PRID=1600895

[27] Carrasco FR, Schmidt G, Romero AL, *et al.* Immunomodulatory activity of <I>Zingiber officinale</I> Roscoe, <I>Salvia officinalis</I> L. and <I>Syzygium aromaticum</I> L. essential oils: evidence for humor- and cell-mediated responses. J Pharm Pharmacol 2009; 61(7): 961-7. [http://dx.doi.org/10.1211/jpp/61.07.0017] [PMID: 19589240]

[28] Kim SH, Lee YC. Piperine inhibits eosinophil infiltration and airway hyperresponsiveness by suppressing T cell activity and Th2 cytokine production in the ovalbumin-induced asthma model. J Pharm Pharmacol 2009; 61(3): 353-9. [http://dx.doi.org/10.1211/jpp.61.03.0010] [PMID: 19222908]

[29] Bui TT, Fan Y, Piao CH, *et al.* Piper Nigrum extract improves OVA-induced nasal epithelial barrier dysfunction *via* activating Nrf2/HO-1 signaling. Cell Immunol 2020; 351: 104035. [http://dx.doi.org/10.1016/j.cellimm.2019.104035] [PMID: 32051090]

[30] Shukla S, Bajpai VK, Kim M. Plants as potential sources of natural immunomodulators. Rev Environ Sci Biotechnol 2014; 13(1): 17-33. [http://dx.doi.org/10.1007/s11157-012-9303-x]

[31] Gheware A, Dholakia D, Kannan S, *et al.* Adhatoda Vasica attenuates inflammatory and hypoxic responses in preclinical mouse models: potential for repurposing in COVID-19-like conditions. Respir Res 2021; 22(1): 99. [http://dx.doi.org/10.1186/s12931-021-01698-9] [PMID: 33823870]

[32] Johnson TS, Narayana DBA. Role of spices in offering natural immunity to fight various diseases. Pharmacogn J 2020; 13(2): 600-13. [http://dx.doi.org/10.5530/pj.2021.13.76]

[33] World Health Organization. WHO guidelines on safety monitoring of herbal medicines in pharmacovigilance systems 2004. https://apps.who.int/iris/bitstream/handle/10665/43034/9241592214_eng

[34] Mohammadi N, Shaghaghi N. Inhibitory effect of eight Secondary Metabolites from conventional Medicinal Plants on COVID_19 Virus Protease by Molecular Docking Analysis. ChemRxiv 2020. [http://dx.doi.org/10.26434/chemrxiv.11987475.v1]

[35] Vimalanathan S, Ignacimuthu S, Hudson JB. Medicinal plants of Tamil Nadu (Southern India) are a rich source of antiviral activities. Pharm Biol 2009; 47(5): 422-9. [http://dx.doi.org/10.1080/13880200902800196]

[36] Amber R, Adnan M, Tariq A, Mussarat S. A review on antiviral activity of the Himalayan medicinal plants traditionally used to treat bronchitis and related symptoms. J Pharm Pharmacol 2017; 69(2): 109-22. [http://dx.doi.org/10.1111/jphp.12669] [PMID: 27905101]

[37] Gilani AH, Khan A, Raoof M, *et al.* Gastrointestinal, selective airways and urinary bladder relaxant effects of Hyoscyamus niger are mediated through dual blockade of muscarinic receptors and Ca^{2+} channels. Fundam Clin Pharmacol 2008; 22(1): 87-99. [http://dx.doi.org/10.1111/j.1472-8206.2007.00561.x] [PMID: 18251725]

[38] Hussain F, Jahan N, Rahman K, Sultana B, Jamil S. Identification of hypotensive biofunctional compounds of *Coriandrum sativum* and evaluation of their Angiotensin-converting enzyme (ACE) inhibition potential. Oxid Med Cell Longev 2018; 2018: 1-11. [http://dx.doi.org/10.1155/2018/4643736] [PMID: 30581531]

[39] Khan MY, Kumar V. Mechanism & inhibition kinetics of bioassay-guided fractions of Indian medicinal plants and foods as ACE inhibitors. J Tradit Complement Med 2019; 9(1): 73-84. [http://dx.doi.org/10.1016/j.jtcme.2018.02.001] [PMID: 30671369]

[40] Mishra S, Aeri V, Gaur PK, Jachak SM. Phytochemical, therapeutic, and ethnopharmacological overview for a traditionally important herb: *Boerhavia diffusa* Linn. BioMed Res Int 2014; 2014: 1-19. [http://dx.doi.org/10.1155/2014/808302] [PMID: 24949473]

[41] Rege AA, Chowdhary AS. Evaluation of Ocimum sanctum and *Tinospora cordifolia* as probable HIV protease inhibitors. Int J Pharm Sci Rev Res 2014; 25(1): 315-8.

[42] Nair R. HIV-1 reverse transcriptase inhibition by *Vitexnegundo* L. leaf extract and quantification of flavonoids in relation to anti-HIV activity. J Cell Mol Biol 2012; 10(2): 53-9.

[43] Thayil SM, Thyagarajan SP. Methanol and aqueous extracts of *Ocimumkilimandscharicum* (Karpuratulasi) inhibits HIV-1 reverse transcriptase *in vitro.* Int J Pharmacogn Phytochem Res 2016; 8: 1099-103.

[44] Ganjhu RK, Mudgal PP, Maity H, *et al.* Herbal plants and plant preparations as remedial approach for viral diseases. Virusdisease 2015; 26(4): 225-36. [http://dx.doi.org/10.1007/s13337-015-0276-6] [PMID: 26645032]

[45] Khanna K, Kohli SK, Kaur R, *et al.* Herbal immune-boosters: Substantial warriors of pandemic Covid-19 battle. Phytomedicine 2021; 85: 153361. [http://dx.doi.org/10.1016/j.phymed.2020.153361] [PMID: 33485605]

[46] Petr D, Marian H, David V, *et al.* Anti-inflammatory and antitumor promoting effects of the triterpene acids from the leaves of *Eriobotrya japonica.* Nat Prod Rep 2006; 23: 394-411.

[47] Augustin JM, Kuzina V, Andersen SB, Bak S. Molecular activities, biosynthesis and evolution of triterpenoid saponins. Phytochemistry 2011; 72(6): 435-57. [http://dx.doi.org/10.1016/j.phytochem.2011.01.015] [PMID: 21333312]

[48] Ding S, Jiang H, Fang J. Regulation of immune function by polyphenols. J Immunol Res 2018; 2018: 1-8. [http://dx.doi.org/10.1155/2018/1264074] [PMID: 29850614]

[49] Ververidis F, Trantas E, Douglas C, Vollmer G, Kretzschmar G, Panopoulos N. Biotechnology of flavonoids and other phenylpropanoid-derived natural products. Part I: Chemical diversity, impacts on plant biology and human health. Biotechnol J 2007; 2(10): 1214-34. [http://dx.doi.org/10.1002/biot.200700084] [PMID: 17935117]

[50] Sengupta PS. Use of Piper Betel to combat COVID19. PREPARE@ U- Preprint. 2020.Available from. [http://dx.doi.org/10.36375/prepare_u.a92]

[51] Lu S, Strand KA, Mutryn MF, *et al.* PTEN (Phosphatase and Tensin Homolog) Protects Against Ang II (Angiotensin II)-Induced Pathological Vascular Fibrosis and Remodeling—Brief Report. Arterioscler Thromb Vasc Biol 2020; 40(2): 394-403. [http://dx.doi.org/10.1161/ATVBAHA.119.313757] [PMID: 31852223]

[52] Olafsdottir ES, Ingólfsdottir K. Polysaccharides from lichens: structural characteristics and biological activity. Planta Med 2001; 67(3): 199-208. [http://dx.doi.org/10.1055/s-2001-12012] [PMID: 11345688]

[53] Gaikwad MS, Meshram BG, Chaugule BB. On the occurrence of the genus Porphyridiumnageli: new to India. J Algal Biomass Util 2009; 1(1): 102-6.

[54] Winston D, Maimes S. Adaptogens: herbs for strength. Stam Stress Rel 2007; (Apr): 226-7.

[55] Pike JW, Christakos S. Biology and mechanisms of action of the vitamin D hormone. Endocrinol Metab Clin North Am 2017; 46(4): 815-43. [http://dx.doi.org/10.1016/j.ecl.2017.07.001] [PMID: 29080638]

[56] Erol A. High-dose intravenous vitamin C treatment for COVID-19. Ind Res 2020; 1: 1-7. [http://dx.doi.org/10.31219/osf.io/p7ex8]

[57] Liang Y, Wei P, Duke RW, *et al.* Quantification of 8-iso-prostaglandin-F2α and 2,3-dinor-8--so-prostaglandin-F2α in human urine using liquid chromatography-tandem mass spectrometry. Free Radic Biol Med 2003; 34(4): 409-18. [http://dx.doi.org/10.1016/S0891-5849(02)01018-3] [PMID: 12566066]

[58] Mastaloudis A, Leonard SW, Traber MG. Oxidative stress in athletes during extreme endurance exercise. Free Radic Biol Med 2001; 31(7): 911-22. [http://dx.doi.org/10.1016/S0891-5849(01)00667-0] [PMID: 11585710]

[59] Huang Z, Liu Y, Qi G, Brand D, Zheng S. Role of vitamin A in the immune system. J Clin Med 2018; 7(9): 258.

[http://dx.doi.org/10.3390/jcm7090258] [PMID: 30200565]

[60] Kang EJ, Kim SY, Hwang IH, Ji YJ. The effect of probiotics on prevention of common cold: a meta-analysis of randomized controlled trial studies. Korean J Fam Med 2013; 34(1): 2-10. [http://dx.doi.org/10.4082/kjfm.2013.34.1.2] [PMID: 23372900]

[61] Mousa HAL. Prevention and treatment of influenza, influenza-like illness, and common cold by herbal, complementary, and natural therapies. J Evid Based Complementary Altern Med 2017; 22(1): 166-74. [http://dx.doi.org/10.1177/2156587216641831] [PMID: 27055821]

[62] Fuhrman J. Immunity benefits of Zinc as we age. Very Well Health 2020; 27: 1-3.verywellhealth.com/surprising-immunity-benefits-of-zinc-4047431

[63] Spritzler F. 2018.https://www.healthline.com/nutrition/10-foods-high-in-magnesium#section7

[64] Rayman MP. Selenium and human health. Lancet 2012; 379(9822): 1256-68. [http://dx.doi.org/10.1016/S0140-6736(11)61452-9] [PMID: 22381456]

[65] Ivory K, Prieto E, Spinks C, *et al.* Selenium supplementation has beneficial and detrimental effects on immunity to influenza vaccine in older adults. Clin Nutr 2017; 36(2): 407-15. [http://dx.doi.org/10.1016/j.clnu.2015.12.003] [PMID: 26803169]

[66] Kalra EK. Nutraceutical-definition and introduction. AAPS PharmSci 2003; 5(3): 27-8. [http://dx.doi.org/10.1208/ps050325] [PMID: 14621960]

[67] Kanauchi O, Andoh A, AbuBakar S, Yamamoto N. Probiotics and paraprobiotics in viral infection: clinical application and effects on the innate and acquired immune systems. Curr Pharm Des 2018; 24(6): 710-7. [http://dx.doi.org/10.2174/1381612824666180116163411] [PMID: 29345577]

[68] Roy A, Sarkar B, Celik C, *et al.* Can concomitant use of zinc and curcumin with other immunity-boosting nutraceuticals be the arsenal against COVID-19? Phytother Res 2020; 34(10): 2425-8. [http://dx.doi.org/10.1002/ptr.6766] [PMID: 32488956]

[69] Manoharan Y, Haridas V, Vasanthakumar KC, Muthu S, Thavoorullah FF, Shetty P. Curcumin: a wonder drug as a preventive measure for COVID-19 management. Indian J Clin Biochem 2020; 35(3): 373-5. [http://dx.doi.org/10.1007/s12291-020-00902-9] [PMID: 32641876]

[70] Shrivastava R. Immunity boosters: Solutions from nature – Herbs and spices. Journal of Renal Nutrition and Metabolism 2020; 6(2): 35-7. [http://dx.doi.org/10.4103/jrnm.jrnm_20_20]

[71] Kumar V. Seven spices of India—from kitchen to clinic. Journal of Ethnic Foods 2020; 7(1): 23. [http://dx.doi.org/10.1186/s42779-020-00058-0]

[72] Girija PLT, Sivan N. Ayurvedic treatment of COVID-19/SARS-CoV-2: a case report. J Ayurveda Integr Med 2020; 20: 30042-5.

[73] Arshath Jyothi PS, Dileep A, Devarajan D, *et al.* Three case reports of moderate COVID-19 infection managed through Ayurvedic approach. Journal of Ayurveda Case Reports 2020; 3(3): 84-90. [http://dx.doi.org/10.4103/jacr.jacr_57_20]

[74] Ang L, Lee HW, Choi JY, Zhang J, Lee MS. Herbal medicine and pattern identification for treating COVID-19: a rapid review of guidelines. 2020. [http://dx.doi.org/10.1016/j.imr.2020.100407]

SUBJECT INDEX

A

Sachin Kumar Jain, Ram Kumar Sahu, Priyanka Soni & Vishal Soni (Eds.)

B

F

G

K

L

M

N

O

P

R

S

T

W

Z

Made in the USA
Las Vegas, NV
03 November 2026

57424146R00119